'Tis t

A Collection of Reader-Submitted Medical Stories

Kerry Hamm

Disclaimer:

Names, locations, and portions of the details included in this book have been altered to protect the privacy of those involved.

<u>**Warning:**</u>

This edition features light profanity that may be offensive to some readers. The profanity has been used sparingly and in each instance the usage was included in the submission. I have chosen to leave some of these words in to emphasize portions of the stories.

By now, I am sure you are all too familiar with my *Real Stories from a Small-Town ER* series, which were collections of stories told to you from my time as a registration clerk in Ohio. If you are new here, don't fret! You don't have to worry about a 'certain order' for *any* of my books, including this one!

I have since moved on from the hospital scene, but that hasn't stopped readers from submitting stories of their own experiences from the medical field. Over time, I have received hundreds of stories-some funny, some sad, some downright scary or grotesque-and have worked with my readers to bring these stories to you in a follow up to my last *Real Stories* volume.

If I've learned anything from writing my series and compiling this book, it's that none of us are alone. We're all proof that we've seen some seriously messed up things out there, right? We have seen the good. We've seen the bad. We've seen the downright vile and disgusting. And then, we've seen the humor in these situations and we've been fortunate enough to share them with one another. There is a certain peace in knowing that as no matter how crazy we feel, we have formed solidarity amongst ourselves, knowing that for every bad day you've had, others have had them too. We have worked through the challenges of getting up and facing another drug seeker, another child abuse case, another young death, and another 'how the heck did that even happen?' moment together. You guys are not alone, and this book reaffirms that.

Several of the stories have been edited to bring you clear-cut and clean versions of tales submitted by loyal readers. I have done my very best to edit out hospital and town names, and in some cases my submitters wished to withhold their initials and other details from publication or requested that I edit stories for grammar/spelling. Some stories have been edited for length. I do my very best to preserve a reader's humor and emotions, as well as capture the reader's personality when I edit these submissions.

Though some of the stories in this collection are horrifying, I am glad none of us are alone in what we've witnessed or experienced.

<u>Cheat Sheet</u>

Some readers have been confused about terms used in this series. Here's a quick list to help you out!

LEO: Law Enforcement Officer

ETOH: shorthand for Ethyl Alcohol or Ethanol; commonly used to describe intoxicated individuals

Bus/Rig/Truck: Ambulance

M.D.: Medical Doctor

R.N.: Registered Nurse

MVA: Motor Vehicle Accident

EMS: Emergency Medical Services

EMT: Emergency Medical Technician

PD/FD: Police Department/Fire Department

D.A.: District Attorney

BOLO: Be on (the) Lookout

DCFS/CPS: Department of Children and Family Services/Child Protective Services

SNF: Skilled Nursing Facility. This can be a nursing home or facilities for patients in need of supervised care

AMA: Against Medical Advice

A Christmas Miracle

Back in the late-1980s, I was one of
three ES registrars scheduled to be on shift
at a large hospital located just outside a
major city. One of my coworkers called in
sick, and the other went into active labor
while she was registering a patient, so I
was left alone until help could arrive. It
was so busy that patients waiting to be
registered were lined up from my work
station to the sidewalk outside. Back in
the day, nursing and clerical staff operated
on different software systems, so nobody
could help me. One nurse saw how
stressed out I was on this insanely-busy
evening shift, and she brought me a cup of
coffee strong enough to wake the dead.

I did not have an opportunity to drink
that coffee, however, because no matter
how many patients I registered and sent to

the waiting area, eight more would arrive. During that time, I was cussed out, yelled at, and threatened. The hospital employed one security guard per floor back at that time, and as luck would have it, our floor's security guard was assisting someone else. That always seemed to happen when I needed him.

Until the end of time, I will keep this memory in my mind. Because our information desk was closed early, I was attempting to assist a family in finding their daughter's room. The problem with this is that none of them spoke English, so I was losing my mind from trying to figure out a way to tell them that she had been transferred to an inner-city hospital with a NICU wing.

While this family continued growing frustrated and shouted at me, a man staggered inside, followed closely by two women. They were dressed nicely, with the man in a suit (no jacket), and the women both in tight business skirts, ruffled tops, and kitten heels.

"We need some help!" one of the women shrieked. "Please, can anyone help?"

I was already on the phone, calling for medical assistance. Nobody had to tell me twice.

What had thrown these ladies into panic mode was that they were following the man closely, so they could support the artificial Christmas tree branch coming out of his lower back. He was impaled through and through by a green metal bar that appeared to have entered through his lower back and was fully visible through a hole in his lower abdomen.

From that second on, everything happened so quickly. I remember the family at the desk had still been yelling at me, so I pointed a finger to the row of seats along the wall and recall screaming, "Sit down and wait." I know they didn't understand my words, but they seemed to understand the urgency of the situation around them, so they all were seated. Two nurses and a doctor from the ES treatment area arrived to the front with a gurney and made the impaled patient lie on his side as they wheeled him back. A nurse asked the ladies accompanying him if they could give his identifying information, and between the two of them, we registered the patient with just his name, date of birth, and verifying that he was the correct 'John Smith' by only the name of the street on which he lived. I then informed the women to be seated and someone would come for them when the patient was allowed visitors. The two were trembling and crying. I noticed one woman's hands were covered in blood, so I escorted her to our patient wash station and allowed her to clean up.

Back at the front, as I was inspecting the lobby and foyer floors for blood, the family from the row of seats bombarded me again, and I could see my coworker walking across the parking lot to enter for her shift.

"I can't understand you, and you can't understand me," I said to them. I held up my index finger. "If you give me one minute, I can try to contact someone. I don't know what language you're speaking. I'm sorry."

Other patients flooded in to be seen, and I returned to my station. The family searching for their daughter followed me and cut off other patients so they could get to the front of the line. They continued to yell at me, and the patient's father slammed his palm on the counter and screamed the patient's name.

"I can't translate anything for you!" I shouted, immediately turning red because I lost my temper. I took a deep breath and said, "I don't know what language you're speaking."

I was almost crying when I pleaded with this family, in a language they couldn't understand, to take a seat. Patients behind them were growing angry.

"It's Cantonese," someone chimed from the back of the line. "Do you need help translating?"

I stood and saw a middle-aged woman pushing an elderly man in a wheelchair.

"Honey, do you need help translating?" she asked again, as tears finally started making their way down my cheeks.

I nodded, and she left her father in line as she approached my work area. With her help, we informed the family that their daughter had been transferred. We all apologized to one another, and the family left. I couldn't thank that woman enough for her assistance.

With my coworker's help, we managed to register all the patients from the line, and then I worked on discharging patients as she continued to work on active charts.

The two ladies from earlier approached the desk and asked if I had an update on the patient they'd brought in. I called to the unit clerk and was informed the patient had been transferred to emergency surgery approximately 15 minutes ago. When I called the surgical unit clerk, she checked on the surgery process and informed me that they could not give me an update, other than the man was in stable condition and the length of the surgery was unknown because his internal injuries were unknown. I relayed this information to the women, and they cried.

I shouldn't have asked what happened, but my curiosity got the best of me. The women explained the three worked together at an office a few blocks away. They had stayed late to decorate the office for Christmas. While the women were working on piecing together the artificial Christmas tree, their male coworker was standing on a ladder, hanging garland. He fell off the ladder and landed on the base of the Christmas tree. The metal rod went right through him. These ladies said they removed the branches from the bottom portion of the tree before driving the man to our hospital.

For four hours, these women waited in a crowded room filled with sick patients, and they never complained to me once. One of the women disappeared down the hall and returned with two cups of hot chocolate from our new vending machine. She gave the beverages to my coworker and me, saying she thought we deserved the kind gesture. It did not go unappreciated.

Someone from the surgical wing met the women and brought them to a consultation room just behind my work station. I could hear the male nurse as he explained to the women that the metal rod had missed every vital organ in the patient's body. There would still be a cause for concern over the ligaments and muscles in the man's back, but for now everything appeared to be in good shape. The nurse stated everyone was surprised and could consider this nothing else but a miracle.

I heard this again when the women left the consultation room and came to share the good news. I saw the ladies a few more times over the following weeks, as they came to visit their coworker during his recovery. They were the only visitors he had. When the patient's health took a turn for the worst and he contracted an infection, the women arrived and stayed for two days straight, forgoing showers, and living off food from the cafeteria and vending machines. My coworker told me that one of the women talked to her in the elevator and said that the man's girlfriend had died earlier that year, right after his mother had passed away. Neither woman wanted to leave the man alone for the holidays, especially after he hurt himself. I always thought that was a kind gesture.

The patient was discharged on Christmas Eve.

--K.W.

California

On New Year's Day, I registered a woman for head pain. The patient said she had been violently vomiting, when she jerked forward and smacked her head on her toilet bowl. She also requested treatment for her hangover.

X-rays showed a hairline fracture on the woman's frontal skull. She literally fractured her skull by hitting her head on the toilet as she was vomiting.

If that's not the definition of a bad hangover, I don't know what is.

--A.S.

Michigan

I Must Be the Way God Intended

J.S. from Wisconsin submitted this gem. Most of his submission remains exactly as written. He has a real knack for storytelling!

I work nights for a private ambulance company that has a 911 contract with the city fire department to respond to emergency medical calls. I'm an EMT, so we operate as a basic life support unit responding to calls that are non-life threatening and don't require IVs, Advanced Medications, heart monitoring, or treatments of the sort.

My partner, in her late thirties, was working her last shifts before her new job started. She'd usually work eight hours on a weekday day shift. She, too, mostly encountered non-emergency transports and discharges between facilities. This was the first night shift she'd worked at our company since training, and she had so far been baptized by fire. We'd responded to a car accident, had several drunk patients, and almost, **almost** had to help a new mom deliver a baby in the back of the ambulance. I'd been working nights for all but the first month of my career and my usual partner was a bit of a black cloud, so I was used to the insane pace.

Seven hours into the cold overnight midwinter shift, with no break yet and none in sight, dispatch sent us to a call in one of the poorer neighborhoods right on the edge of our service area. Our dispatch monitor read: **Nature**: "Other – See Comments." **Comments**: "May be asleep." Dispatch further advised us "Police are Aware."

Lovely.

When we arrived on scene, my partner flipped on the emergency and scene lights, illuminating the figure laying on the sidewalk with the ambulance's floodlights. I got out and knelt next to the patient. I shook his shoulder and asked, "Hey man, are you alright?"

Our patient was wearing an oversized dirty jacket, filthy blue jeans, and a hoodie underneath the jacket. When I shook his shoulder, he opened bloodshot yellowish eyes and screamed, "AHHHHHHHHHHH!" as he leapt to his feet.

I swear, he didn't even use his hands to scramble up from the ground. I had jumped back, too, and I could smell enough ETOH rolling off him to supply a pub.

He wildly screamed again, "I AM SATAN!"

My partner and I exchanged a bewildered expression.

"I'll get the cot." said my partner, showing enough common sense for both of us.

"I AM SATAN!" The patient screamed again, rattling windows up and down the street.

"Okay, Lucifer" I responded, "Have you done any drugs tonight?"

"Yes," he said. He then started taking deep, rapid breaths.

"Which drugs did you take?"

"I took ALL THE DRUGS!"

I guess I left myself open for that. He made the last part a yell and shrugged out of his coat, dropping it onto the sidewalk.

My partner rolled the cot to the curb stood next to me, saying to the patient, "How about you take a seat on the…"

"I MUST BE THE WAY GOD INTENDED," howled the patient. Before

I knew what was happening, this guy was pulling off his hoodie.

"Hey, man" I said. "How about you hold on a second. It's pretty cold out…"

"I MUST BE THE WAY GOD INTENDED!"

He tossed his hoodie aside and stripped from his equally-filthy tee shirt. Next, he undid his belt and dropped his pants, exposing his boxers. I've been in this field for quite some time and it's hard to faze me anymore, but I must admit, this patient was a bit too much for me.

"Maybe we should leave the pants on." I said weakly.

My partner, again showing enough common sense for all of us, keyed up her portable radio and asked for an ETA on the Police.

The patient ignored us and, without wobbling or falling or kicking, got his jeans off over his sneakers. That's probably the single most impressive thing I've ever witnessed another human do, especially drunk and high. I wondered if he'd had practice.

The patient then dropped his boxers, exposing everything. He pulled off his boxers, twirled them over his head, and threw them into the wind. They hit the side of the ambulance and bounced into the snow.

He screamed; "I AM THE WAY GOD INTENDED!"

Wearing only his shoes, the man bolted from the scene, balls flapping into the night, as he sprinted down the street.

"Should we follow him?" my partner asked.

I carefully watched as the patient crossed out of our service area and into the service area of a different ambulance company.

"No." I said. "Now he's PD's problem."

"Won't we get in trouble for losing a patient?"

Though I was also worried about that, I tried not to show it. After all, we weren't supposed to follow crazy patients, right? Instead of engaging in a foot pursuit with our naked runner, we put the cot away and then called dispatch. I put the phone on speaker, so my partner and I could both hear what dispatch was saying. Since I knew the dispatcher, I was elected to explain the situation. I intended to divvy out some intelligent butt-covering report, but when I heard "Dispatch," I blurted everything out at a mile a minute.

"Hey, this is Ambulance 15. Our patient just fled the scene…naked."

If you're familiar with dispatchers, you know they're on the ball, all the time. Nightshift dispatchers are like the Hulks of dispatch: they're rarely fazed, they get right down to business, and they try to have your back. So, without missing a beat, the dispatcher asked, "Okay, which way did he run so I can notify PD?"

You'll Shoot Your Eye Out, Kid

A young male patient received a BB gun as an early Christmas present and was soon rushed via ambulance to our ER because the pellet he fired ricocheted off the chain link fence post and hit his eye.

As many young patients do, the child cried and squirmed, making examination almost impossible. He was bleeding all over the room, and he just wouldn't stay still. Having his mother in the room did nothing in keeping him still.

Finally, we were able to calm the patient and we examined his eye. He sustained a deep corneal abrasion and complained that he could not see out of that eye. The wound was not severe enough that the patient would lose his eye, but the doctor worried that the patient would permanently lose his eyesight due to the accident.

The patient's father arrived, and this guy was a hoot. His idea of 'helping' during this time of stress for his child and wife was replying to his family and our staff by only using lines from *A Christmas Story*—that movie TBS is always playing on a loop on Christmas Day.

Though the patient's wife was fuming and accusing him of not caring enough about their son's health, we couldn't keep ourselves from laughing. One of our physicians, who is a real hard-ass that none of us like because I don't think he's so much as broken a smile in 13 years, laughed so hard that he had to excuse himself from the patient's room. The patient had gone from sobbing to laughing hysterically. Mom was the only one who was mad.

By the time of discharge, the patient announced some of his eyesight had returned. We were later updated and learned that the patient retained limited eyesight in the affected eye, but he would suffer forever from a 'blind spot' where the pellet had hit, meaning for the rest of his life he will see a black spot.

--D.I.

Illinois

Cold as Ice

Our hospital accepts volunteers to fill the position of escorts. These volunteers guide visitors through our large hospital so that we don't have frustrated family members or friends wandering around for hours, trying to find a patient. We pride ourselves in accepting only the kindest, most patient volunteers.

One of our volunteers was a teenager with Down Syndrome. He was such a sweet soul who loved making people smile. He'd go out of his way to assist visitors, and he was a doll. Sometimes, if a visitor was upset, John would take money from his own pocket and buy the visitor flowers from the gift shop or coffee from the cafeteria. Everyone loved him.

We had this jerk come in one day, and he was a real class act. He was the

31

stereotypical 'business type' you see in movies, the kind of guy who couldn't waste a single second of time, who was incapable of saying anything nice to anyone, the kind of guy who screamed orders at anyone he thought was beneath him—and you know the type; everyone was beneath him.

He came to the information desk when the secretary was in the restroom, and I could hear him screaming from all the way in my office, which was down the hall. He kept yelling the name of a wing that we don't have assigned in our facility. Then he started screaming a man's name, saying he needed to find the patient.

When I emerged from my office to offer assistance, the man was yelling at John, who was taking the verbal beating in stride.

The man waved his arms around as he turned in a circle and he screamed, "Does this place have anyone except retards working here?"

John was calmly trying to explain to the man that the secretary would be back momentarily, and she would be able to use the computer directory to find the patient. John explained this would only take a moment, and then the man could be on his way.

Still, the man screamed. He called John a retard to his face, and then he continued to belittle John, telling John his parents should have had him aborted.

Absolutely disgusted by this man's behavior, I marched down the hall and gave him a piece of my mind before we both realized he had come to the wrong hospital. He stormed out, never once apologizing to John or to me for his vile display.

Some time passed, and a rough snow storm was passing through. John was the only volunteer who made it in to escort visitors through the facility, but since it was snowing so heavily and we were not receiving enough visitors to need an escort, we thought it would be best to send John home before the storm worsened. He was visibly upset but understood and thanked us for our concern over him walking back to his home.

A few minutes after John bundled up and left, I heard him shouting for help. I bolted from my office and saw John carrying a man over his shoulders like soldiers do on the battlefield. John was crying and said the man was lying in the parking lot, covered in snow and sleet.

A team from the ER came down and took the man away. I was so caught up in the commotion and busy trying to calm down John that I didn't get a good glimpse at the patient. I had to call John's mother because he was so emotional that I couldn't get him to just breathe. I'd never seen him like that before, and it was troubling, to say the least.

John complained that he was hurt, too, so we walked to the emergency room and registered him as a patient. We later found out that John pulled a muscle in his back and dislocated his right shoulder in the process of bringing the patient inside.

The patient wanted to meet the man who saved his life and John went to the patient's room.

No fooling, it was the man with the nasty attitude we had encountered weeks earlier. He had recognized the signs of a heart attack and drove himself to the nearest hospital. He passed out in the parking lot, and nobody would have even known he was there if John hadn't been leaving early. John happily gave the patient a hug.

It sounds outrageous, but I think maybe it was the universe's way of telling that patient to extend compassion and respect to everyone.

Unfortunately for us, John moved away with his family a few months later.

--E.M.

New York

We registered 18 patients for knife-related injuries between Christmas Eve and New Year's Day last year. These injuries were strictly related to the holidays and excluded domestic or gang violence. All 18 patients stated they had either cut or stabbed themselves or others while attempting to open gift packaging.

Calm down out there, guys. That Magic Bullet blender isn't worth a $3,000 hospital bill.

--T.H.

New York

It Happened One Christmas

I am a nightshift nurse, so I generally get back home around 07:30, unwind for a few minutes, and sleep from 08:00 to 12:00. I get up to see the kids home from school/make dinner/help with homework, and then (if I can) nap before work. The kids had Winter Break and my husband was home, so I had an entire week of sleeping through the day. I can't tell you how excited I was. You really don't know the value of sleeping without interruptions until you have to split your rest.

On this day, especially, I was thrilled to sleep in. The snow was coming down hard and fast, and we were supposed to get about six inches by nightfall. My neighbors plowed our road and the side streets so we could get to a main road, so I always loved waking up to see all the snow.

I don't know if I just couldn't stay asleep because I was excited about the weather or my mom-alarm kept telling me I needed to go check on the kids, but I tossed and turned for about four hours before I finally fell into a deep sleep. It was the kind of sleep where you start dreaming as soon as you close your eyes.

That lasted about five minutes. I woke to the sound of breaking glass, followed by a loud thump, followed by my youngest kid screaming her head off. Seconds later, my other two kids were screaming. And then, my husband started yelling, "Oh, no. Oh, I don't know what to do."

When I stood at the top of the stairs and looked down the steps, the house was a disaster. There were Cheerios on the stairs like breadcrumbs leading Hansel and Gretel through the forest, someone had spilled a cup of milk on the hall floor and *left* it there, and there were toys all over the place.

That's not even the half of it.

There were three air mattresses stacked on top of one another, that took up most of the living room. The television was knocked over and hanging off the stand. The ceiling fan light was broken, and there were shards of glass everywhere. My husband's foot was bleeding and he was trailing blood all over our brand-new $700 carpet. Both of his hands were bloody as he held them against my youngest daughter's head in two places. My other kids were standing on the couch. One of the cats was sitting in the corner, looking confused about what was going on. The dog was standing out on the patio, covered in snow and whining, with her nose pressed against the patio window.

I was more interested in checking on my injured kid than knowing what happened, but I found out anyway. You know how kids in commercials are all sweet and innocent and polite and charming? Mine aren't. As soon as they saw me descending those stairs, my two oldest started tattling on my husband and injured kid. Of course, they *swore* they not been involved, which I already knew was a boldface lie because I know my kids.

From what I could gather, my idiot husband was running out of ways to keep the kids busy indoors, so he went through our camping gear and blew up the air mattresses for the kids to jump on like a trampoline. I'm still not sure which genius came up with this part, but the kids would lie flat on the top mattress and my husband would then belly-flop on it, sending the kids up in the air. I guess nobody used math to figure a 34-pound toddler catapulted into the air by a 214-pound man would go flying much higher than anticipated. My daughter hit her head on the ceiling fan light so hard that she broke it, hit her head on the edge of a chair when she landed, and my husband cut his foot open on glass as he ran across the room to check on her.

Oh, I was steaming. I was beyond-words angry. I was exhausted because the previous night was a full moon and we all know how those suck the energy right out of you. I knew that night wouldn't be any better, especially if I couldn't get any sleep.

We couldn't even get out of our driveway because of the way it's sloped, and the snow had fallen, essentially blocking us in. We had to call one of our neighbors and he was nice enough to come out in a hurry to plow the road and drive us to a main road in his tractor, so we could meet an ambulance. His wife stayed with my older kids while my husband and I were at the hospital.

I felt so dumb when we got to the ER because after my daughter was cleaned up and we got a better look at her wounds, her lacerations were so superficial that I probably could have handled it myself…if I had not been freaking out, at least. My daughter had to get two stitches and I requested a CT scan just to be on the safe side. My husband needed three stitches to close the cut to his foot. He cried more than my daughter did when it was his turn to be sewn up.

We were in the ER for four hours to do all that, and getting home took another hour. I had to help my husband clean up all the mess and my neighbors wanted to talk about what had happened, so I ended up calling in, using a personal day. I was upset about that, too, because I was one of six people in the entire hospital who'd not called in that year, and at the end of the year we were going to split a prize package that contained money, gift certificates to restaurants and a spa, and vouchers to be used at Ticketmaster.

It's been a while since this happened, but I still bring it up pretty much every chance I get. I don't know what my husband was thinking. I know it was an accident, but it was almost like I left a teenager in charge. Even with insurance, we had to pay $1,200 out of pocket for the ER visit, and we had to pay $300 for a company to come out and clean our carpet. We also had to buy a new ceiling fan.

We now have a new rule: no jumping on air mattresses in the house.

--J.G.

Wyoming

Baby, It's Cold Outside

Imagine this: you've just worked for 22-hours straight because there was a nasty storm that rolled through your rural town, pelting roads, vehicles, and everything in sight with fat raindrops. Now imagine that sometime during these 22-hours, a cold front came through, freezing everything that was wet from the rainstorm. Then imagine responding to at least two dozen MVAs. Imagine the frustration of knowing you only have minutes to respond to reports of an infant turning blue from possible choking, but you can't take the rig over 20 MPH without running the risk of sliding right off the slick streets and putting your truck out of service for the unforeseeable future. Imagine a baby dying in her mother's arms, while a five-year-old watched the whole thing because he got out of bed to see what the commotion was. You don't get the luxury of relaxing. You don't get to take a nap. You can't cry on the way back to the station because it's your turn to drive.

And as soon as you find yourself a block away from that station, moments from a 12-year-old mattress that's beat up and uncomfortable and doesn't fit you, but it's a place to lie down to try to get rid of your splitting headache and upset stomach, you hear dispatch calling your rig for assignment. It's also 03:40.

I have a love/hate relationship with my dispatchers. On that night, I hated the guy on shift. I complained that we were tired; he said, "John, we're all tired." I guess I shouldn't have been mad at him. He was right.

I've heard people say that sleep deprivation does the same thing to your body as when you're drunk. I can testify to that. On the rig, I was in a mood, one that I could have used to conquer the

46

world. Then I felt loopy, but a tired loopy, where my head bobbed, and my partner couldn't ask if I was okay to drive because he was asleep in the back, lying on the cold, muddy floor as I was hitting every bump and pothole possible, just to try to stay awake.

I don't think dispatch put us on the call due to our proximity. They put us on the call because I used to run this place. Literally. I was a camp director at this little patch of land a few miles out of town, where we'd take kids for the summers and teach them things like how to make a fire or how to patch a pair of jeans. We tried to make it educational *and* fun. For fun, we'd jump into this huge lake that was a mile or so from our campsites.

That's why dispatch sent me there. He knew I'd be more likely to navigate this area that had become a teenage hangout after the camp shut down two decades earlier. Maybe I shouldn't have told you that. I'm showing my age.

My partner woke up after I punched him in the arm.

"Gotta walk from here," I said to him.

He groaned, "Why?"

"Only thing getting through that field is an ATV. Do we have an ATV?"

"Why can't we just find a road?"

"Because the roads weren't maintained and were overtaken by weeds. Come on, gotta walk from here."

"So, if this girl has a broken leg, we gotta carry her?" he asked.

I nodded and said dryly, "Looks that way."

"I'm gonna kill Bob," said my partner, threatening the dispatcher.

"I won't have the energy," I said. "As soon as we transport this patient, I'm clocking out. I don't even care what they say. I need to rest before we run again."

"Agreed."

We continued our conversation as we made the four-day trek across the vast lands of ice. Just kidding. It was about five minutes of walking until we reached the frozen-over lake. There was a girl lying on the ice, crying.

"Help me!" she screamed. "I'm over here."

My partner started to rush forward, but I stopped him.

(If you use my story, make sure you let everyone know I said this *heroically*.) "I gotta do this," I told him.

"Why's that?"

"I'm lighter," I said.

"So?"

"So?" I mimicked. "Look, the ice isn't trustworthy right now."

"Well, it's not like I was going to tell it my deepest, darkest secrets," my partner snapped.

I pointed to spots around the shore and used my flashlight to motion down the lake. "See that discoloration?"

He nodded.

"It's not frozen through. Don't come out on the ice. I'm going to get her and bring her back to shore, if I can."

I dropped my bag and eased out on the ice. It was solid from what I could tell, but I didn't trust it since I'd noticed we were maybe 10 feet from weak ice. I could tell you a thousand stories about weak ice, but that's not what this one is about.

When I approached the patient, who couldn't have been a day over 20, I kind of stood over her and gave her a weird look. Out of nowhere, it started raining, as in cats and dogs.

"What the hell happened to you?" I asked.

She was lying in an awkward position. Her right leg was straight, as she rested mostly on her flat back, but her left leg was pulled upward into an upside-down/lopsided triangle, with her foot by her head.

"Please help me," she cried. "I'm so cold."

She may have been a little warmer if she wore something more than leggings and a thin hooded shirt, but what do I know?

"Can you stand?"

She cried, "If I could stand, I wouldn't have called 911."

"Touché," I replied. "What's hurting the most?"

"My leg," she said. "It's been in this position for, like, 20 minutes before I called you."

And then I saw why.

The patient's ice skate blade had become entangled in her long hair. When she went for the twirl, the blade snagged, and she went down. She told me she had tried to get the hair untangled from the blade, but she couldn't, meaning she couldn't move.

I laughed and laughed and laughed. I swear, it wasn't because I'm this hateful person. I was tired. You could have showed me a picture of a single black dot at that moment, and I would have still thought it was hilarious.

She and I both went dead-silent when we heard a loud crack beneath us.

I had no choice but to move her, even though she complained of leg pain. We could feel patches of the ice moving under our feet as I moved her off the ice.

As men, my partner and I didn't exactly have a lot of experience with female hair. The patient begged us not to cut her hair loose, so we transported her to the ER. I think a few smart nurses were able to get most of the hair untangled by smothering her hair in conditioner, but we were later told that 'some of the hair just had to go,' and they snipped away tangles they couldn't relax.

The girl's only significant injuries were a dislocated hip and a concussion.

--G.A.

Michigan

Untitled

This is one of those cautionary tales.

I was in charge on the night a man was brought in for injuries he sustained in a sledding accident. He had been out drinking for hours with his friends, when they decided it would be a good idea to go sledding. The men did not own a sled, so they stole the lids off garbage tins from a group of homes near the park.

The group of three, at two in the morning, raced each other down a snowy embankment. They stated they did this several times with minor injuries (a male from the group was treated for two broken fingers).

Unfortunately, one of the trips downhill went terribly wrong.

One of the men slid into the roadway and was hit by oncoming traffic.

His injuries included fractured ribs, internal bleeding (including a ruptured spleen), so many contusions that a good part of his face and arms were nearly black, multiple lacerations, and severe head trauma.

This man was rushed to surgery from A&E, where skilled and dedicated surgeons worked for hours to save his life. Unfortunately, following surgery, the patient developed a secondary brain bleed and experienced swelling. He died the next morning.

If I could tell my patients one thing, it would be this: do not mix alcohol with ideas like this. When you're intoxicated, you are not making safe decisions, and though this is the worst-case scenario, I have personally witnessed injuries that could have been avoided if someone with the ability to make proper choices had been included.

This man passed away two days after Christmas, and I cannot imagine the suffering his family and friends endured or must endure during each holiday.

--S.T.

'A traveling nurse in Europe'

<u>Babes in Toyland</u>

My partner and I were dispatched to a complaint in sexual nature, but we were given little more to go on than 'patient is stuck.' We didn't know what to expect, honestly. I remember it was NYE and all night we'd been running MVAs and things related to alcohol, so this call stood out.

When we arrived at the apartment building, the doorman let us in and we took the elevator upstairs. This woman was standing in the hallway, wearing this almost-transparent robe. She hurried us inside and was talking excitedly about how she and her girlfriend were 'experimenting' and then 'they made a mistake.' She said something about 'we don't know how to get them off.'

Oh boy.

When we entered this dark bedroom, there was a woman on the floor, with her feet in these black leather straps that held her legs behind her head. And on her mouth...holy crap. I didn't know what it was at the time. It looked like a torture device, honestly. This woman's lips were squeezed between this metal grid thing that looked like a waffle fry. Like, her lips were all swollen and smashed between these bars that were locked on her mouth. Then I realized that her tongue was also in the device, smushed. (I found out later the device was called a tongue and lip press. It's basically a locking device that squeezes the user's tongue and lips between clamps, and the whole thing is made out of steel.)

The woman who was all confined in this stuff, she was crying. I don't know if she was scared or hurt or embarrassed, but I imagine it was a little bit of each. Her girlfriend knelt and showed us that the locking mechanisms on the straps and the clamps were 'stuck,' and the patient had been in the devices for approximately 40 minutes already.

I'm going to be honest here. I had no idea in holy hell where to even start with this stuff. I mean, you can tell from my descriptions that I didn't even know what these devices were.

My partner, this scrawny, nerdy, quiet type who hardly talked about anyone—and when he did, it was religious-talk—he knelt down and said, "There's a little button here. You have to press it as you're pulling on the belt. It's to keep the straps in place during use."

That surprised the hell out of me and everyone back at the station.

It took us a minute to figure out the mouth clamps, but once we managed, my partner muttered, "Hmm, maybe I should order one of these."

We left the apartment after the patient and her girlfriend thanked us and assured us they'd be more careful in their future experiments.

Since that day, I've never looked at my partner the same. I guess it goes to prove that it's the quiet ones that have the most fun.

--M.W.

Utah

Last Christmas

We were contacted by a female concerned about her father's wellbeing. He was known locally for his Christmas spirit, as he displayed lights on his house year-round and left his porch decorated the same. He even had an inflatable snowman in the yard, during winter, rain, or unbearable summer heat. The caller stated she hadn't heard from her father in nearly a week, following an argument revolving around the daughter's work schedule and her inability to make it to the traditional family Christmas dinner.

When we arrived at the residence, everything appeared to be in order on the outside of the house. Lights were in working order, decorations were intact, and nothing seemed out of place.

I rang the doorbell, which chimed a holiday tune.

No answer.

I then knocked.

No answer.

I walked around to the back of the house and knocked on the back door. It was there that I had a view of the home's interior and saw a chair tipped over on the floor. My gut told me this did not seem right.

I forcefully entered the residence. This man loved Christmas and anything to do with it. His kitchen had a North Pole theme, with candy-cane-striped washcloths and oven mitts. The man had those plastic decal things in windows, and he even sprayed fake snow in all the windowsills. He had Christmas decorations in every room.

I found this gentleman hanging in the doorway between the dining room and the living area. He had constructed a noose out of thick rope and was hanging, all while dressed in a festive holiday sweater and nice slacks. The holiday lights he had placed around the doorframe from which he was hanging were turned on and twinkled to the tune of music playing from another room.

I found it difficult to break the news to the man's daughter. We discovered shortly after finding his body that the man was diagnosed with cancer and it was thought he would not survive to have another Christmas. I'm not sure if the medical team was supposed to tell us that, but we kept our mouths shut as to not further upset the man's daughter. She found out, anyway, because her father had written her a letter and mailed it before hanging himself. She was a mess (understandably) at her father's funeral, and we all felt horrible for her family.

--L.M.

Minnesota

*Author's note: If you are considering harming yourself or just want to talk, help is available. Call the National Suicide Prevention Hotline at 1-800-273-8255.

Silver Balls...Errr...Bells

We received at least a dozen complaints about a 'lewd' snowman on someone's front yard.

First, when we arrived, we saw there were technically two snowmen. One was a woman, on all fours. The second was a male figure behind her. Use your imagination here. It was definitely what many would consider an inappropriate display.

I laughed. Sorry, not sorry. Still, as an officer, I have to set aside my personal feelings and act in the interest of the public. Many of the callers were parents who were complaining that a K-8 school bus traveled the area daily, and children had begun asking questions about the creative display.

I knocked on the front door of the home and was met by an older man, probably in his early-60s. Right off the bat, I was thinking the guy's son or grandkids probably constructed the snowmen.

"Sir," I said, "we've gotten a few complaints about the artwork on your front lawn. Now, I think it's wonderful that your kids are out here playing, but maybe we can come to an agreement to knock this one down and let them build something a bit more...ahem...family friendly."

The man seemed confused. "No kids made that. I did. And if I want to build a snowman of a woman pissing on my front lawn, I'll do that next. That's why it's called *my* lawn. Now take your complaints elsewhere."

He then slammed the door in my face.

I knocked again.

"Go away," I heard him yell.

I rang the doorbell.

He swung that door right open and yelled, "Didn't I tell you to go away?"

I shook my head. "Sir, look. Personally, I think this whole thing is ridiculous and I find your artwork humorous. But others don't. They're worried about the small children seeing it."

"Kids see worse than that just going to school," the man argued.

I agreed. "But I have a job to do, and we can't have that kind of art displayed for the whole town to see."

"I fought for my rights," the man protested. "If I want to sit on my lawn naked and read a *Hustler,* by God, I'm going to do it."

"Sir, that's not quite sure how far freedom stretches," I said with a chuckle, "even though we've all probably had the idea cross our mind a few times."

No matter how relatable I tried to seem to this homeowner, he wasn't having it. Finally, I just told him, "Look, I'm going to have to cite you if it's not removed in an hour. I don't care how you do it. I don't care what you put in its place, as long as it's not lewd or disruptive. I think it's funny, but a lot of other people don't, and I have to respond to those complaints."

"Charge me with what?" the guy yelled.

I was at loss for words. Well…I didn't know. They were snowmen. It wasn't like he was the one on the lawn engaging in sexual activity.

"Just have it removed. You have an hour. I'll be back to check."

The man slammed the door in my face again and I left.

At the shop, we discussed between us what kind of charge this would warrant, if the homeowner chose not to remove the piece. We couldn't charge him for indecent exposure because he wasn't exposing himself. We decided that this was similar to someone showing someone a *Playboy* in the alley. I guess it could have been stretched to sexual aggravation, but we settled that it would fit best under disorderly conduct because his artwork was disturbing the peace.

Of course, an hour later, the piece was still there.

I knocked on the front door again, and the man opened the door.

"I'm not taking it down," he said.

"Then I'll have to cite you for disorderly conduct."

"You're going to arrest me?"

I shook my head, "That wasn't my plan. I was just going to write you a ticket.

If you want to keep fighting me on this, though, it could lead to an arrest. I'm trying to work with you here, I really am."

The man snatched his jacket from his coat rack and stomped through the front yard.

While he was kicking, punching, and digging at the sculpture, he was screaming and cussing loudly.

"Aren't you going to arrest me?" he yelled. "I'm saying bad words, officer!"

I laughed. "You're allowed to be angry. As long as you plan on stopping soon, I'm not doing anything to you."

After the homeowner finished destroying his artwork, he apologized to me and invited me in for a beer. I had to decline his offer because I was on duty, but told him I'd take a raincheck. I understood his frustration. We seem to live in a world where we can't say or do anything because all humor is lost on people who take issue with every little thing. I can't make a joke about stepping on a cat's tail these days because some animal activist will chime in and tell me that's considered animal abuse and that's not funny. No, animal abuse isn't funny, but sometimes jokes are. Sometimes a joke doesn't mean you agree with the actions performed in it or that you're a horrible person...most jokes are just jokes because they're funny. This homeowner's art display was lewd, and yes, I could understand the complaints from neighbors, but I empathized with his viewpoint on his freedom and how far we had to take this.

It didn't take long for the homeowner to sculpt another snowman. We received complaints on this one as well, with callers threatening to tear down the piece because it 'was violent and pressured children to react violently.' The new sculpture was a traditional three-snowball snowman, draped in an old military blouse and cap, waving an American flag.

We saw nothing offensive, disturbing, or illegal about the second sculpture, so we spent hours arguing with callers that the homeowner was well within his rights to display this snowman. Our homeowner called once to complain that his sculpture had been vandalized and someone had stolen the military jacket from the sculpture. On his second call, he complained that someone had destroyed his snowman and placed a sign next to the flag stating if he chose to display one flag, he should display them all. We never caught anyone, and we didn't have any suspects.

I'm still shaking my head over all of this.

--D.L.

Ohio

Merry Christmas, Everyone

The day after Christmas, we had a patient come in for 'emergency tattoo removal.' He said he went out with the boys, had one (or 12) too many, and visited a tattoo shop. Now hungover, he was incredibly concerned about his young children viewing the disturbing artwork, and he was afraid his ex-wife would be able to use the artwork against him in their custody dispute.

Across his chest and abdominal region was a depiction of Santa ejaculating on a 'sexy' elf's behind, while Mrs. Claus engaged in intercourse with multiple elves. In the background, an elf was performing sexual activities on what appeared to be a reindeer.

I had to explain to the patient that the Emergency Room does not perform tattoo removal, and I suggested he seek out a professional removal service. Until then, I told him, to keep his shirt on and stop drinking.

The patient stayed for hangover relief and asked for something to help with his anxiety over the tattoo.

We saw him again the next week; his tattoo had become infected.

--J.M., M.D.

Florida

All I Want for Christmas Is...

We were having one of those nights that we were calling a 'Psych/Bed Night,' when most of our patients were homeless, mentally ill, or both. These patients were registering because they needed counsel or a bed, which I'm sure you could figure out. It had snowed four inches in just a few hours, and some of these people simply had no place else to turn.

Now, I see so many mentally ill patients that these people can say or do the craziest things, but I just don't laugh (during or after) anymore. I guess I've let reality hit me of how bad off some of these patients are, and these days I feel more sad than able to find humor in situations.

On this night, though, something happened that had me laughing so hard that I peed my pants. I'm ashamed to admit that, but all my coworkers saw, so I guess there's no point in trying to hide details of what happened.

A patient came to the registration area to check in with our clerks, and I was scrolling through the computer to pull the next patient by priority of complaint.

I guess the patient had already registered and was just coming in from a smoke break to ask how much longer it would take. This person obviously had a problem because he looked disheveled and talked to himself. At one point, he was talking to a coat rack. He just wasn't 'all there.'

"We'll call you as soon as we can get you back," said the clerk. "Go ahead and take a seat, please."

I didn't pay too much attention to the man as he disappeared into the waiting room, but I did hear security shout, "Hey!"

When I looked up, they were chasing the man through the foyer. He was carrying a chair from the waiting room.

The patient looked like a deer in headlights as he spoke with security.

"She told me to take a seat," the man shrieked wildly. "I'm just as confused as you are!"

Soon, tears were streaming down my face and pee down my legs. I had to walk through the busy ER to get to my locker for another pair of scrubs, so about 10 nurses, 3 doctors, maybe 3 or 4 registration clerks, and God-knows-how-many patients saw that I had an accident. Everyone started asking me if I was okay, and I was still laughing so hard that I couldn't reply.

I was laughing for the rest of the night, and when I think of this patient, I start laughing out loud again.

--M.T.

New York

The Christmas Box

One year, we treated a male patient for second and third-degree burns to his face, chest, neck, and arms. His injuries were serious, and he required sedation.

We learned the patient had presented his wife with a Christmas gift. When she opened it, she was angry to find sexy lingerie. It wasn't the lingerie she was mad about, though. The lingerie was not her size, and she found the card inside addressed to another woman. Her husband accidentally gave his wife his girlfriend's Christmas gift.

In a fit of rage, the man's wife flung a pot of boiling soup at him. Not only was he burned by the liquid, but he was also burned when hot vegetables stuck to his skin (he had a piece of potato practically stuck to 'melted' skin). He passed out from shock. I guess his wife called 911 and admitted what she'd done, and she was arrested when officers and medics arrived.

We had to fly the patient out to a facility better-equipped to treat his injuries. I have no idea what happened to him after that. I mean, I understand how angry that wife must have been, but I can't imagine being so angry that I leave someone disfigured.

--M.N.-E.

Arizona

Here Comes Santa Claus

Back in the mid-1990s, we had a report from a convenience store clerk that a man dressed as Santa had robbed her at gunpoint. He had fled on foot.

We didn't think we had a snowball's chance in hell of catching this guy because Christmas was a week away and there were people in Santa suits on every corner, collecting donations for one charity or another.

Our plan was to drive around the back block of where the convenience store was located, hoping the guy would be there. We were then going to travel down a side street, passing the front of the convenience store, before traveling to the block in front of the store. We didn't think he could have gotten more than two or three blocks away if he didn't have an accomplice acting as a getaway driver. Maybe, just maybe, we thought, we would spot a Santa who just didn't fit in.

Nothing seemed out of place behind the convenience store. As we drove down a side street and neared the front of the store, we saw something that stood out: one Santa Claus was standing against the brick building, with three children surrounding him. We noticed the plastic bag in his hand right away. This was our guy.

As soon as he saw our car, he took off. It was unfortunate that it happened this way, but we deployed a taser on the subject…in front of those three kids. As soon as we managed to fight the kicking, screaming, and foul-mouthed Santa to our car, I felt so badly about what happened that I had to take a moment to approach the young children and tell them that the man we had arrested was a man pretending to be Santa, and we were taking him to jail.

The kids were so young that I'm not sure if they really understood anything that was happening. I still think about them today and wonder if this instance made them stop believing.

Anyway, we took the imposter to jail and someone asked why he stopped to talk after he just robbed a store. He said, "They're kids, man. What kind of heartless bastard do you think I am?"

--P.E.

Illinois

<u>You're a Mean One...Mr. Grinch?</u>

A few years back, we took a report of some missing gifts a wife who claimed on three or four gifts had gone missing from under the family's Hanukkah Bush. She was 'positive' neither her kids nor husband removed the gifts, and furthermore, she stated her back door had been ajar when she had woken. We filed the report, but there wasn't a lot we could do. The caller couldn't remember what gifts she had wrapped in those packages, and we didn't have hard evidence that someone outside of the home had been the culprit.

The next morning, the husband called, telling us a similar story. Again, I asked the husband if his children could have taken gifts, to which he replied, "They know better."

We took another report, but again, we couldn't do much. We offered to beef up patrol in their neighborhood for that night, but none of our patrolmen reported suspicious activity near the residence.

On the third morning, we still received a call. The wife stated three more gifts were missing and she knew this because she counted the gifts before going to bed. She said she confronted her children, both whom denied stealing and were in tears by the time their mother ended an interrogation.

This woman reported she had also confronted her neighbors, and she thought the easiest way to gain a confession would be accusing first instead of asking. None of her neighbors had stolen from the family, and now she had fewer friends in the neighborhood.

The complaints annoyed me. It was frustrating because we couldn't help them much, but we knew there was going to be another complaint in the morning if we didn't do *something*.

Again, we agreed to patrol the area, but we also decided to take one of our guys and park him in the alley behind the house, since the back door was reportedly left open in two of the three complaints.

Our patrolman radioed the station at 03:00 and was laughing so hard we couldn't understand anything except, "Call them. Tell them to go behind the garage."

We didn't know how to explain this to the family, but we assured them it was safe and our patrolman would accompany the husband and wife, once he stopped cackling.

Our patrolman witnessed the family's yellow lab emerging from the back entrance, carrying a wrapped gift. He reportedly took the gift behind the family's garage, before he headed back to the home two more times for another load of gifts. Behind the garage, the family and the patrolman found the pupper's stash. There were 14 gifts there, mostly still wrapped, except for small gashes as a result of the dog's teeth or the weight of the gift slipping from the paper during transport.

Also found in the stash were remote controls, socks, a pair of keys, newspapers, and magazines.

We recommended to the family that they secure their home and/or the dog at night, to prevent this in the future.

--J.U.

Idaho

Be Good for Goodness' Sake

I may be a horrible person for finding the call we responded to funny, but I couldn't stop laughing once we wrapped up all six arrests.

I guess our local mall was responsible for holding district-wide job interviews for several positions of 'North Pole Elf,' that were reportedly paying $9 an hour, which was good money then. We learned approximately 18 positions were open for potential applicants. More than sixty applicants arrived for open interviews.

When we arrived on scene to the 'all available officers' dispatch, the scene was hectic. About 20 individuals, mostly little people (and, oddly enough, one 6 ½-7-ft-tall man wearing green tights under booty shorts and a tunic top), were brawling. Most of these individuals had dressed the part of a North Pole elf, so essentially, we had a bunch of Santa's elves beating the crap out of each other in the storage room of the mall. Bells on costumes were jingling, individuals were screaming, items from the storage area were flying through the air. One individual had grabbed a broom and was beating another applicant with the handle. Two people had to go to the hospital for wounds sustained in the fight.

It took a while to get everyone settled. We took reports from bystanders and from some of the calmer subjects. We came out of there with three possible reasons the fight began, but they weren't related. There were three separate fights going on when we had arrived.

This happened before the days of putting mugshots online, and I bet most of our subjects are thankful that they're not floating around the Internet in work attire.

Like I said, I'm probably going straight to Hell for thinking it was funny, but I'd never seen anything like it except in movies, and I never thought I, of all people, would respond to a call like that.

Most of the subjects got off easy because they were first-time offenders, but we did find one had open warrants.

--H.M.

Colorado

Die Hard

A homeowner's security system was triggered and the company notified us, as the homeowners had notified the security company of going out of town for the holiday. (Advice from an officer: you can call most security companies and they can make a note of this; if your company practices this, call them before you leave. It will cut down on response time and potentially save your valuables and time.)

When we arrived at the residence, we figured the perp was long gone. After all, we could hear the alarm system blaring from the sidewalk. (Remarkably, not ONE neighbor was awake to check on this residence, and we received NO concerns or complaints from callers.) Surely, nobody would be thick enough to remain at the residence, right? You'd think someone would hear the alarm and run, right?

While my partner was working with dispatch to have the alarm company silence the alarm, I moved through the home and turned on the living room lights. A man jumped up from the couch and pointed a gun at me.

Now, I wear a vest, but that vest isn't going to protect my head, arms, or legs. And I've been shot before; just because you have that vest on, doesn't mean you're not going to feel it. I've been shot while not wearing the vest and can tell you I'd rather be shot while wearing it, but it doesn't mean that it's a fail-safe when dealing with an armed subject. The point here is that I didn't want to be shot.

"Put your weapon down," I shouted.

"No."

"Put your weapon on the ground now," I repeated.

"No."

"I don't want to have to shoot you," I informed the man.

He smiled, and I'll never forget that face. He said, "But I want you to."

Unfortunately, this wasn't the first attempted assisted suicide I have encountered. Though the first encounter I had ended badly (the subject shot me in the shoulder and another officer returned fire, killing the subject), I had made it up in my mind within five seconds of this man telling me that, that I wouldn't let it all end that way, not again.

For a few minutes, we continued screaming orders and answers at one another, but then I tried to reason with him by telling him about my life and asking him about his. He was ready to die, but I wasn't ready to kill.

"So," I said, "I have three kids. Been married eleven years. What about you? Any kids? Got a woman?"

He shook his head. His hand was shaking. "Have an ex. She got a good lawyer and got custody of the kids. Better to pretend they don't exist, since I'll never see them again."

"That's a shame," I said. I tried to relate to the subject by saying, "The system really screws over dads, doesn't it? I have a kid from a fling. Haven't seen my son since he was born."

That was a lie, but he didn't know that. I thought the guy was going to come around, but when I asked if we could talk without weapons drawn, he began screaming again. This talk-down, get worked up thing went on for about another five minutes.

My partner moved from the hall to the doorway. I didn't realize he had even moved from the hall, he was that quiet.

In a half-second, the subject fired his weapon. My partner went down. I had to use that moment to return fire. My brain never told me that I had any other option to disarm the subject. It happened so quickly, but when I dwell on the memory, it replays in slow motion. My conscience nags at me, telling me I had ample time to take the subject down with a tackle or stun gun or any kind of non-lethal force. Mandatory counseling sessions with a therapist who told me I did what I could at the time helped a little, but I know I'll probably think about this for the rest of my life.

It may sound like it, but the subject didn't die. I shot him in the leg.

A lot of us still go through the motions, even if we only wound a subject. I did what I had to do, I know that. My partner lived. If I hadn't had returned fire, neither my partner nor I would probably be here today. I think this really bugs me because this man *wanted* me to kill him, and I simply can't understand being in the state of mind where I could be so uncaring of someone else's mental health to pressure them to commit that act. I don't blame the subject. I know he was in a bad place.

Now, I haven't spoken to the subject since this night, but I did hear he was receiving the help he needed…from behind bars.

A few good things came from this: my wife is always a lot more *giving* when I'm involved in such an incident; my kids stopped screaming at each other for about an hour before they picked up again; my partner bought me tickets to go see my favorite band, and I got a guy off the streets without killing him.

--T.Z.

Washington

*Author's Note: I can't be the only one thinking this man deserves a raise, right?!

P.S. Die Hard *is* a Christmas movie. Let's put that argument to rest. ;)

Nightmare Before Christmas

Christmas Day dragged on. We had seen three patients over a span of six hours, so most of our time was spent listening to music, snacking from the carry in food, and some of us had either gone to the waiting room or empty patient rooms to watch television.

Two police cars pulled up to the ER entrance and I returned to the registration desk, where the male clerk made a joke that the cops were probably just as bored as we were and were coming to steal our food.

The first set of officers entered with a woman who was holding an ice pack to the back of her head. She had been crying and she had two black eyes and a broken nose.

The second set of officers entered with a man who had lacerations to his face and hands. He was also bleeding from the nose and appeared to be missing a tooth. He was wearing only a pair of house slippers and a pair of flannel pajama pants.

I watched as the clerk registered the first patient. She only stated, 'head injury' as her complaint and did not further elaborate.

The male refused to speak to the registration clerk, so the officers gave the patient's name and further information.

This man, having spent too much time on the internet, read about a possible way to heighten the pleasure of an orgasm. He and his girlfriend (the female patient) engaged in sexual intercourse, in which the female was on all fours. During this time, the boyfriend punched the female in the back of the head, which caused her face to slam against the nightstand adjacent to the bed. Her nose broke on impact.

Upon realizing her boyfriend had performed what the internet calls a 'Donkey Punch' (Google at your own risk), the female hit him in the face with a lamp she had grabbed, and when he hit her as retaliation, she then grabbed a fireplace poker and wacked him again.

The female patient was treated and released. She worked with officers to file for an emergency restraining order against her boyfriend.

What I found funny here, as in funny-outrageous, not funny-ha-ha, is that the male in this situation was screaming that he wanted the female arrested for assaulting him. Can you believe that?

Some of us closely followed the case via details released from the officers who responded that day, but we didn't hear much, except the male was arrested for assault and the female was granted an order of protection.

Personally, I think this guy got what was coming to him for abusing an innocent girl. Imagine him having to call his family or friends on Christmas Day and explain why he needed bail money!

--C.V.

Indiana

If you are involved in an abusive relationship, help is available. Call the National Domestic Violence Hotline at 1-800-799-7233.

<u>Can You Hear What I Hear?</u>

About 20 years ago, the city saw a string of assaults and one murder on female joggers/walkers. Most of the victims had reported rapes or other sexual assaults, as well as were transported hospitals for lacerations, contusions, and even broken bones. One jogger had been reported missing by her mother. Her body was found the next morning, tossed in the bushes like litter.

As you can imagine, fear ran rampant. Our officers did not want to feed into this panic, but we also didn't want to ignore that we had a person or persons out there, harming females just trying to relax or exercise.

Our Chief at the time gave a statement to female joggers to carry a whistle, be alert of surroundings, play music at a volume that was quiet enough in headphones to still hear if anyone approached, avoid the area at night, and if possible, visit the area with a friend or group.

I have a wife and daughter now, and some of that is good advice, but I'm going to tell you what I've told my 26-year-old multiple times.

When you hear a car alarm outside, what do you do? If you hear a whistle or noise from a block away, what do you do? What do most of us do?

That's right, we think, 'Hmm, someone's alarm is going off,' or, 'Someone's making a lot of noise.' We tell ourselves that the car's owner accidentally pressed the alarm button and will shut it off momentarily. We hear that voice in our heads telling us that someone's kid just got a whistle as a toy.

Be honest here: how many of you investigate that noise?

Now, I'm not telling you to go out as a crimefighter in a robe, only to become a victim yourself.

But like I also tell my daughter, a cell phone isn't going to help you none if you someone busts you in the face and you can't reach your phone to not only dial 911, but also give dispatch your location.

I know we all have these notions that it's safer to go out in daylight, but the truth is, I've reported to just as many assault complaints during the day as I have at night, if not more. These people aren't afraid of the sun. They pick their locations based on the density of bystanders, so going in a group or with a friend is actually good advice.

Being aware of your surroundings is always good advice, as is being alert. Unfortunately, that doesn't always work out in your favor. You're not always going to listen to your gut. Sometimes your gut isn't going to tell you that something doesn't seem right. There have been serial killers who were able to convince women to help them load furniture by climbing into a van and then killed those women. There are times you're going to think you're doing the right thing because that's going to be your natural reaction to a situation, but that assailant is *hoping* you react that way because he's already devised a plan.

Now, I'm going to tell you how the string of assaults and one murder ended way-back-when, before I offer more advice.

One female's husband bought her a 116-pound American Bulldog-mix from an ad in the newspaper. She had owned the dog for two hours, when she decided to take him on a walk in the area that the assailant frequented.

This woman, despite having a huge animal companion at her side, was violently attacked. Her assailant punched her in the head and knocked her to the ground. Before he could drag her off the walking trail, however, her dog lunged at the assailant and bit his arms, face, and neck. While the dog was attacking the assailant, the female was able to make it to a payphone and call for help. Her new dog was still attacking the assailant when I arrived on scene. Unfortunately, the dog died because the assailant had stabbed the dog multiple times during the attack. This dog died a hero.

There was so much blood in the snow that, as the new kid on the block, I was assigned to find a hose and melt the snow from the trail. It took half an hour to melt the snow and wash away the blood.

The point in all of this is that you must always be prepared. Always. Carry a weapon that you feel you can control. If you don't feel comfortable carrying mace, don't do it until you feel you're ready. Contact local authorities if you're unsure if a particular weapon is legal to carry. There are a variety of devices out there, cloaked to look 'cute' and non-threatening if that is what you prefer, but they actually pack a punch, such as keychains that double as stun guns or a sort of stabbing device. You can purchase mace, knives, or firearms (never carry unless you are familiar and comfortable with firearms and are licensed) that may be concealed. If you do not feel comfortable carrying a weapon, contact your local college or police station to learn if there are self-defense courses nearby. In no way do I mean to sound like I'm victim-shaming, but there are also cosmetic ways you can keep yourself safer. Wear comfortable, but practical clothing. Can you run in heels? Will your flip flops hurt someone if you need to kick? You shouldn't *have* to change your appearance to go running in the park, but maybe consider wearing your hair in a bun instead of a ponytail that an assailant can use to yank you back and drop you to the ground. Always tell someone where you're going and how long you think you'll be.

Over the years, I can't tell you how many assaults on walkers or joggers I've responded to, but even one is too many. Nobody should ever have to feel unsafe while exercising or enjoying leisure time. Hopefully, though, my tips can help someone find empowerment and avoid being another victim.

--H.S.

Then New Jersey, now Delaware

Grandma Got Ran Over by a Reindeer

We were already at the town's Christmas parade as standby medics, when we witnessed a frightening accident.

The parade lineup passing us was comprised of a firetruck, a police car, and two horse-drawn carriages. The first horse-drawn carriage carried our Santa and Mrs. Claus. Following closely behind them were Santa's 'elves,' who were throwing out candy from these huge burlap sacks.

Mrs. Claus stood from her carriage and attempted to lean over the side to toss one of ten 'special' wrapped gifts to a small child standing on the sidewalk. You can probably guess what happened next.

Yes, she fell over the side.

This woman's dress somehow became caught up on something on the side of the carriage, and she rolled under the wagon. Before anyone could signal the following driver to stop, three horses stomped on Mrs. Claus.

The scene was chaotic. Parents forced their children to turn around. Kids and adults were crying and screaming. The driver of the second carriage kept apologizing. It took five minutes for the lineup to pull up enough for the second carriage to move from the location, while Mrs. Claus laid underneath, crying out in pain.

This woman was extremely fortunate. She suffered from a collapsed lung and fractures to several bones, including her hips, legs, arms, and facial region.

Throughout our assessment and transport, this woman was in great spirits. She laughed about the situation, despite her collapsed lung, and she expressed concern about the children who'd witnessed the accident.

As Mrs. Claus was healing, she accepted visitors and mail from kids in the locale, who were concerned about her condition. Her priority wasn't her own health, but making sure these kids knew everything would be fine, and helping them in hopes of lessening their traumatic memories.

She laughed off the incident after spending weeks in the hospital, and she went right back to volunteering as Mrs. Claus during our town's next winter parade—where carriages were fitted with seatbelts and standing was restricted.

--S.W.

Utah

Joy to the World

My partner and I were part of three teams that had been dispatched to a frat party on New Year's Eve. Calling that many of us out for a party (or to any scene) indicates trouble. On top of that, I hate responding to campus calls. Everywhere you look, whenever you're called, you're going to see at least one drunk or hungover person puking. That's just the way it goes.

At the frat house, that's pretty much what was going on. We learned about 13 members of the frat, their sorority dates, and guests had become ill from an unknown source, which was later to determined to be alcoholic punch that had been spiked with a smorgasbord of prescription drugs that clash with one another, let alone how they react when mixed with enough alcohol to fill a river.

What was unique about this party compared to others I've responded to was that all the females were either nude or only wearing panties. Most of the girls were wearing fabric antler headbands or had cute holly or mistletoe garland in their hair. Partygoers who weren't ill and didn't want the party to die down encouraged everyone to keep drinking and dancing. Two girls, wearing absolutely nothing but these little cut-out stars over their crotches, were pole dancing on the columns in the front room.

I'm a professional, let me say that. I'm also a 24-year-old man, so I won't lie and tell you I didn't notice so many gorgeous women walking around nearly-naked. Still, I tended to the ill patients, naked or clothed, and did my job to the best of my ability.

Two guys from my workplace had to excuse themselves to their rigs because they had become a little too 'happy' with the party taking place around them. A third guy was sent out to the rig by our superior because he also got an erection, only he went off to flirt with partygoers. He was written up and later quit.

Honestly, beside everyone ralphing all over the place and having to conduct a mass transport to the ER, where the nursing staff hated us that night, that's the best call I've ever been dispatched to. I highly doubt I'll ever be called out to anything better.

--Initials and location withheld at request

I know it's an old urban legend-type story, but over the many years I've been a firefighter, we *have* responded to at least two calls of men trapped in chimneys while dressed as Santa Claus.

My advice to anyone out there would be: just don't do it.

--K.G.

Florida

Jack Frost

I don't know what in the hell would possess someone to do this, but I responded to complaints of a male sitting bare-assed on a metal bench in the middle of December. He was masturbating to females who walked by.

When I arrived, the subject refused to 'put it away.' He ignored my orders to stop stroking himself and was going at it wildly, even though it had begun snowing so much that I could hardly see from all the flakes catching on my eyelashes.

I tried to be nice about it, I really did. But when the man stood and ejaculated on my boots, then still refused to follow orders, I maced him, wrestled him to the ground, and cuffed him—while his pants were still down around his knees.

Emergency room test results showed the man did not have traces of drugs or alcohol in his system. We chalked it up to mental illness and due to the subject's disturbing and violent behavior, a physician kept him as a psych hold.

I don't remember what happened to the guy, but I hope I never have to go through that again. Gross.

--E.N.

Illinois

The Nutcracker

Ladies and gentlemen, this story has me cringing, even before typing out the <u>heavily-edited</u> version of this submission. This is the most outrageous submission I've received so far. J.L. from Nebraska writes:

A few years back, I was a sophomore at college and my fraternity had this huge blow-out party since midterms had been canceled due to weather.

Being a bunch of young, stupid kids, we were determined to have the biggest, wildest party in campus history, so we invited anyone and everyone to this eight-room house, and I think about 300 people showed up before the cops came and broke us up.

After most of the crowd left, we were down to about 20 or 30 guys, and there was so much alcohol left that we were like, fuck it, let's just get as drunk and stupid as we can get. We didn't care. The cable and internet were out because of this bad ice storm, so it's not like we had anything better to do.

Well, after like, an hour of doing nothing but shots *after* we'd already been drinking for hours, we started daring each other to do crazy shit, like one guy dared someone to do naked snow angels in the neighbors' yards. Another guy had to drink a glass of mustard.

Someone got the bright idea to call his ex at three in the morning, so that went as well as you'd expect it to. He got all pissed off and stormed upstairs. He returned with this present, and he ripped the paper off the box like he was the Hulk. He said his ex-girlfriend collected nutcrackers, you know, those wooden doll things. But since he wasn't dating her anymore, she wasn't getting the gift.

We were going to put it on the floor and get baseball bats and go all 'Office Space' on the thing, but another guy told us to wait, that he had an idea. He dared another guy to put one of his nuts (testicles) in the doll's mouth, and then someone was going to smash the mouth closed as hard as they could.

At first, the guy who was dared said he wasn't going to do it, but when everyone started calling him a pussy, he said he'd do it, as long as someone gave him money and let him do more shots first. We had $45 between all of us, and the guy did about six more shots of tequila in 10 minutes.

When it was time, the guy stood up and dropped his pants. Another guy got on his knees and opened this doll's mouth so the guy's nut would fit. We counted to three and the guy who was holding the doll used this lever on the back to slam its mouth shut.

Well, the guy with his nut in the doll's mouth screamed like a little bitch and then passed out. He landed on the table where we had all the alcohol, broke the table, and spilled liquor everywhere.

At first, we didn't want to get in trouble, so we just left the guy there, thinking he'd be fine in the morning. But then, another guy's girlfriend showed up, and when she saw the guy passed out with his pants down and a washrag tossed over his balls, she called 911 and told us we were all stupid. Some of the other guys had passed out by that point, but I'm sure she meant them, too.

I was the least-drunk out of all of us, so I had to tell the paramedics what happened, and one of the guys called us stupid, too.

Well, I guess they took this kid to the emergency room and he was admitted for alcohol poisoning. He also had a ruptured testicle that required surgery, but he was so drunk that he couldn't go right away. He had to wait until the next afternoon, when his blood levels leveled out or something. We heard from his ex that he had to have one of his balls removed and the doctors put, like, a metal ball in there or something like that.

One of my girlfriend's friends reads your books and said I should tell you what happened.

*Author's Note: WOW. Just WOW.

Bad Santa

We responded to our local 'North Pole,' a section of our town square that is decorated year-round for Christmas. This area has two 'cottages,' which are small shack-type structures painted to resemble Santa's 'home' and a 'toy workshop.' People take their kids to see Santa, then can pop on over to the workshop to purchase prints of their digital photograph(s), or buy merchandise printed with the picture(s). During Christmas, the place is lit up so brightly that you can see it from Timbuktu, and there's Christmas music playing. We keep some of the lights on during the off-season, mostly to deter vandalism and to keep the spirit alive.

Our complaint that night was about someone inappropriately touching females. We were surprised to learn our suspect was the newly-hired Santa. Three adult females alleged that Santa touched their breasts and/or buttocks when they approached him with their children. One female stated her brother caught the actions on film, so I took that family aside, while my partner waited for Santa's line to dwindle. Surely, we thought, since he could see me standing right outside the shack and my partner right inside, the man wouldn't do anything illegal.

We noticed something peculiar after a few minutes passed. There were two adults in line, neither of whom accompanied children. Still, the first adult approached Santa and sat on his lap.

Santa did his little 'Ho-ho-ho, what do you want for Christmas?' spiel, before the adult female stated, "To go to Jamaica."

Warning bells rang in my head when Santa shook his head and replied, "I ran out of tickets to Jamaica. You look like you could use a cherry soda. Now, take a

picture and go pay in the workshop.
They'll make sure you get your soda."

I'm not sure why this guy thought this
would work. My partner is the K9 officer
with our department and regularly works
with our drug response unit. I don't have
much experience with dealers as much a s
I arrest for paraphernalia, but both of us
knew the man was talking about strains of
marijuana.

We walked over to the workshop and
arrested the female as she made the
transaction for drugs. The photo booth
clerk placed a baggie of drugs behind the
woman's printed picture, which seemed to
cost her about $40 more than anyone else's
picture.

We tried, we really tried, to keep this
situation calm and operating smoothly.
It's difficult to do that when you have to
call for backup, and then Santa decides to
push a kid off his lap and make a run for it.

We had no other choice, except to use a stun gun on Santa. That didn't go over well with all the parents and children waiting and watching, but we managed to arrest five during this debacle.

--J.F.

Massachusetts

Hard Candy Christmas

If you're going to attempt to burglarize a residence, 1.) make sure the homeowners are gone, and/or 2.) arm yourself with more than a giant, plastic candy cane decoration that you took from the front yard.

Our subject sustained two bullet wounds when the homeowner shot him in the shoulder. The owner was also upset that his sidewalk display was left uneven, due to us having to take his candy cane decoration as evidence. I gave him $20 to buy another one.

--Z.Y.

New Mexico

The Dog Who Saved Christmas

I work in a nursing home, and we were attempting animal therapy, by introducing cats and dogs to our environment. Multiple studies have shown animals can lower anxiety and stress levels in patients, among a number of other results. With management's approval, we introduced to our patients two adult cats and a puppy, a yellow lab-mix.

Unfortunately, this puppy was having a difficult time obeying. Despite the company paying for the puppy to go to obedience school, he still refused to obey on command. He would steal from patients and once, he jumped on one of our residents and tore her thin skin. She required medical treatment.

We were trying to find the puppy a good home. None of our staff could take him due to personal reasons, even though most wanted to. The puppy was a good boy, but we thought he needed a more structured environment, one possibly with children or other animals so he could play. He was not aggressive in the slightest; he simply went all ADHD when he was told to do something, and nothing seemed to help.

I was working an overnight shift and admit that I had fallen asleep after doing my rounds. Only one other nurse was on shift, and I'm not sure where she was most of the night.

It was about four in the morning when I felt nibbling on my hand, which was dangling over the side of my office chair. The nibbles soon turned from soft to hard bites, and then I felt a tug on my scrubs top. When I finally woke, I tried to shoo the dog away. He began barking, and I quickly tried to quiet him so he wouldn't wake my patients. He wouldn't stop barking.

The puppy then started biting at my ankles, running toward the back of the building, and stopping, as if he wanted me to follow him. I'm dumb when it comes to these things, so I told him to go lie down, and I was going to check on my patients again.

When I tried to enter a patient's room, the dog ran and jumped up. With his paws on my bosom, he nibbled at my chin, growled, and ran down the hall. He stopped, looked back, and barked repeatedly.

I finally followed the dog. As we neared his dog door, I thought maybe an animal was outside, or maybe his door was stuck and he couldn't get out to potty on the part of grounds we fenced in for him to go in and out. I checked his door, and when I saw it was working properly, I started toward the front of the building again. The dog refused to follow. He excitedly ran in and out, barking the whole time. He did this about five times, before I finally followed him outside.

I stepped out to the dog's kennel and immediately noticed my coworker's body. She was outside the kennel, lying next to the dumpsters, with a bag of garbage still in her hands. I rushed inside and out another door. My coworker was unconscious, but breathing. The snow under her head was bloody, and she was bleeding from her elbow.

I called 911 and the ambulance transported her to the ER.

My coworker said the last thing she remembered was slipping on a patch of ice. Security footage showed she had been unconscious in the snow for approximately 40 minutes. She was treated for hypothermia, in addition to her superficial wounds.

Once I told everyone how this destructive, disobedient, loud nine-month-old puppy alerted me of my injured coworker, management refused to rehome him. Instead of sending him back to obedience school, our facility's owner paid a trainer to visit each day for two weeks, training the puppy in his own environment and making suggestions, such as purchasing new toys for the dog or taking time out of each shift to 'run him tired.' The trainer suggested that the dog's poor behavior was due to him being a puppy in a low-energy environment; he had been looking for an outlet for his own high-energy.

Once we made these changes, we couldn't have asked for a better mascot for our facility.

Since that night, he's alerted staff of two more serious issues regarding patients: one man had fallen out of bed and his bed alarm malfunctioned, and another patient suffered from a heart attack and was not on monitors, so we would have had no idea if it weren't for our what we call our '911 dog.'

--T.A.

Montana

It's the Most Wonderful Time of the Year

I was having a horrible day before work, and once I started my 12-hour shift as a medic, the day turned to night quickly and the powers that be let me know right away that my bad luck wasn't about to go away.

As soon as I clocked in, and I mean right as I tapped the computer mouse over the button, my name popped up on the 'available crew' monitor, and dispatch told me I was needed at the thirteenth MVA of that day. On our way to accident, we called in three other accidents but did not stop for them. The roads were bad, as you could assume by thirteen MVAs. We had to go much slower than usual, and that made it that much more frustrating to make it out of town, to a paved rural road that we were even lucky to get to. If that MVA had been even one mile more outward, I'm not so sure we would have been able to respond without calling a farmer to help clear the path of snow.

When we arrived at the first MVA of my shift, one older woman who stated to our 911 operator that 'it's really not that bad,' was trapped in her vehicle…that was upside-down in a ditch that was at least four-feet deep.

As soon as I hopped out of the rig, all the hairs in my nose froze and my eyes watered from the sheer chill that seeped to my bones. I was wearing long johns under my BDUs, and I was wearing a winter jacket, but I still couldn't keep the cold out.

I was carrying a backboard and C-collar down the hill, when I slipped and went rolling. Well, the word *roll* makes it sound like this was some kind of eloquent tumble, which it was not. It was not eloquent at all.

When I landed, I hit my knee on the vehicle, and I think I spent about a full minute doing that thing where you clench your eyes shut and try not to breathe because you're hurting so badly. To make matters worse, I was covered in snow. And even though I had been outside for about a minute, the tip of my nose and my fingers were so cold that they had begun hurting.

My partner and I were able to remove the patient from her vehicle without needing assistance from the fire department, which was a freaking miracle in itself.

"You told dispatch your wreck wasn't that bad," I commented to my patient.

"Well," she replied, "I didn't die, did I?"

She was a sassy old lady, and I liked her. She made transport to the ER a little better. My knee still hurt, but we completed the transport and were given a location to stage.

On our way to our staging area, we were dispatched to a report of a possible public drug overdose. No other details were available at the time, but we were told officers were on the way as well.

We arrived at the grocery store first, and we could pick out the guy from across the parking lot. It was easy to see him because he was the only person wearing a leopard leotard when it was 20-something degrees outside.

When we got out of the rig, I asked, "Sir, have you taken any drugs tonight?"

He was too busy running barefoot in front of the cart corral to answer me. It was clear he wasn't experiencing the overdose that was called in, but it was obvious that intervention was necessary to remove him from the parking lot. My partner and I decided to try to herd the man away from shoppers until the police arrived. This didn't go so well, and the man continued running back and forth from the cart corral to the automatic doors, where he'd get up in customers' faces and yell absurdities, like, "Did you know I rode a hippo one time?"

When leotard-man saw the cop car approaching the front of the grocery store, he took off across the parking lot. He then hit a patch of ice, went down, and I think everyone who saw him cringed when the back of his head bounced off the pavement, rendering him unconscious.

Yeah, the guy became a medical transport. Yay!

A few more fun things that I dealt with over the shift were: I dropped both rig laptops and broke them (one I dropped in water, the other on the ground; both were open and were destroyed), so my partner and I had to handwrite reports (he was pissed); I started my menstrual cycle while on a call that I couldn't get out of, and I bled through my new pants and had to explain to the 8-year-old girl in the back of the rig (and her grandfather) why I was bleeding; the Tupperware I had grabbed from my fridge wasn't my lunch, but a moldy mess of unidentifiable leftovers I'd made at least a month earlier; I tripped over my own feet and stabbed myself in the leg with my shears (it was a minor wound and I, luckily, didn't need medical assistance); and we responded to a call of a 550-pound patient needed a lift assist, so we had to call another rig for help and the patient was so upset and embarrassed that he called us so many bad names that if I never get called a bitch again, I won't be upset.

The second-to-last run of my shift was pretty annoying, too, and I doubt anyone has told you anything like this.

Officers requested that we transport a patient for a psychiatric evaluation. The patient had been found harming himself and stated he wanted to harm others. He needed treatment for lacerations to his arms and hands. Some of these lacerations were deep and tendons were visible. He had backed himself into a corner in his kitchen, and responding officers didn't want to stun him or have to use force to take him down, so an officer, my partner, and I attempted to talk the man into coming with us.

That didn't go over that well. The patient grabbed a sandwich off the counter and slapped me across the face with a slice of ham. I was uninjured, unless you count having mayonnaise and ham 'juice' in my eye. I was mostly stunned because I was literally hit in the face with a piece of ham. Like, who else can say that?

Finally, we were on our last call. I didn't even care that it was fifteen minutes before end of shift. I didn't care that it was another MVA. I did not care. All that mattered to me is that it was the last call of the shift. And then, I'd get to clock out and start my PTO, lie on the couch in pajamas, watch TV, drink, drink some more, spend quality time with the boyfriend I'd started thinking I didn't have because I work so much, and not have to respond to any call for a whole five days.

My attitude changed quickly. I think it was when we realized the call was out by the park, and everyone in town knows those roads are never plowed. We drove as close to the call as we could, and we could see what appeared to be a motorcycle on the road in the distance. A male was standing in the center of the road, waving his arms.

We walked a short distance and realized the vehicle was not a motorcycle. It was a motorized cart, like the carts you see people riding at Wal Mart.

The male rider did not appear to be injured, but he was certainly drunk.

We managed to figure out that the man had been joyriding from a home about a mile away. I have no clue how he got that cart through all the snow on the road we were on. He said a farmer had plowed the road down the way, but I didn't know if I should take his word for it or not because he could hardly explain anything without telling twelve other stories and almost falling over because he was so intoxicated.

The man told us his foot hurt, and that his wrist hurt 'when he did this,' which was trying to bend his fingertips back to his forearm.

And then the guy fell against me and vomited all over my brand-new, $170 winter jacket. Chunks of vomit were in the part of my hair that had fallen out of its bun and draped over my shoulders. Vomit dripped off me and into the snow.

I'm not going to lie: I vomited. I threw up once during the initial realization of what the man had done, and then I threw up again as I was trying to get my coat off and accidentally splattered puke on my face.

During this time, the patient had decided to sit down in the middle of the road, and my partner suggested that we get moving to the rig. I was so mad and disgusted that I threw my coat in the field. I still don't know if I could have saved it because it looked stained and the smell of alcohol and whatever else was in that vomit was absolutely disgusting. I think, even if I had saved it, I would have smelled the sick on me every single time I wore the thing.

To make matters worse, we loaded the patient up and tried to turn around, but we were stuck. It was already fifteen minutes after our end of shift, or what was supposed to be the end of shift.

My partner suggested that we could probably push the rig just enough to move it out of its tracks so we could leave. It would be quicker than calling for a tow.

Well, when my partner and I got out and were pushing from the front, the patient somehow got out of the back and argued that 'he could help.' He refused to listen when we told him to either step aside or get back in the rig.

We were pushing and pushing, and finally I felt the rig move. When it did, my boots lost traction, I fell forward, and I hit my face on the rig. I broke my nose and had to spend an extra hour and a half in the ER...as a patient.

That's probably been the worst shift I've had in a long time. It's not easy, earning that $10.00 an hour.

--J.C.

Iowa

Blue Christmas

My partner and I responded to a report of a syncope patient on a busy sidewalk just before Christmas. The report was called in by an officer patrolling the area on horseback, and he stayed with the patient until we could arrive.

On scene, my partner was tending to the now-conscious and coherent patient, who said she was pregnant and hadn't had a chance to eat that morning. She refused medical treatment.

As I was shooting the shit with the officer, his horse—who was tied off to a metal bike rack behind me—started sniffing around. I mean this as the horse was sniffing my buttocks and upper thighs, snorting around my midsection, and was relentless. At first, I didn't want to say anything because I just figured that's what horses do. I've never been around them, really, so I didn't want to come off as stupid for asking this officer what his horse's problem was.

Just as we were wrapping up the conversation, the horse reached its head around and jammed its nose into my crotch, before moving slightly and biting my front upper thigh. I was too busy doubled over in pain from being headbutted in the balls to think much of anything, and in the process, I lost my pants. Yep, this horse pulled my pants down in the middle of a heavy-trafficked area. What's worse than that is I had to basically fight him to pull my pants up, because he was so focused on my pocket that he refused to release my pants. Finally, the pocket ripped off and I pulled my pants up. The horse found a package of opened sunflower seeds I forgot I stashed away.

The absolute worst part about this is that I didn't have any clean underwear that morning, so I had to wear a pair of tighty-whities that had multiple holes on the ass. My girlfriend had been nagging at me to get rid of them, but I would've been going commando without them.

I had to register for a work comp injury because the horse did puncture my skin in one itty-bitty spot. I had a huge black and blue bruise the size of my hand by the time I was medically cleared from the hospital.

--T.R.

New York

__What are You Doing with Your Life?__

This isn't holiday-related, but a friend was complaining to me about ICD-10 codes the other day. These codes are primarily used for insurance purposes, and there are hundreds (if not thousands) of them. If you look closely, there are a few out there that leave you to wonder what exactly is going on in these patients' lives. Here are some weird ones:

- Struck by chicken (W61.32)

- Bitten by cow (W55.21)

- Pecked by chicken (W61.33)

- Toxic effect of unspecified snake venom, intentional self-harm (T63.002)

- Art gallery as the place of occurrence of the external cause (Y92.250—Who knew art galleries were dangerous places?)

- Activities involving arts and handcrafts (Y93.D—Put down the wine and step away from Pinterest, Jane.)

- Splinter in the nose (S00.35—There's also a code for 'Splinter in the breast.')

- Accidental discharge of machine gun (W33.03—If you have a

machine gun and think you may accidentally discharge it, you should probably not have a machine gun.)

- Parachutist entangled in object (V97.21—There are times I think parachuting from a plane would be a fun experience, but then I think of stuff like this happening. No thanks!)

- Piano playing (Y93.J1)

- Open bite of vagina and vulva (S31.45)

- Walked into wall (W22.01)

- Bizarre personal appearance (R46.1)

- Underdosing of caffeine (T43.616A—So, this is a thing? Shut up and give me my coffee!)

- Heelies accident (V005.15—Heelies are the shoes with wheels that pop out of the soles.)

- Crushed by alligator (W58.03)

- Failed school exams (Z55.2—Remember the days of only dreaming of going to the hospital for failed exams after your parents whooped your butt so hard you couldn't sit down?)

- Activity, vacuuming (Y93.E3—As if you need another reason to avoid housework…)

- Exposure of ignition to plastic jewelry (X06.0XXD)

- Struck by falling object on passenger ship (V93.41)

- Bitten by squirrel (W53.21XA)

- Cannabis dependence (F12.2)

Polar Express

One year, I was attending what is called a 'Polar Plunge.' If you are unfamiliar with this, participants gather at a body of water, such as a lake, pond, or river during cold weather. Sometimes, ice is still present, but has mostly been cleared from the water. Participants then rush into the water and quickly exit. I've only heard of these events being hosted as fundraisers, but I suppose they have been organized for other reasons as well.

I was not participating in the event. I just like to see the goofy getups people wear (such as scuba headgear or colorful bathing suits). Every now and then, you'll see some crazy frat guy jump in completely naked. It's a hoot to see everyone's reactions as they hit the water or emerge from it. It's also funny to watch these people talk themselves up so much, just to chicken out and stop at the edge as everyone else jumps in.

The first group of people, about 60-70 out of a crowd of over 300, jumped in the water. At first, everything seemed okay. Paramedics were on standby. Volunteers handed out towels and/or bathrobes to people emerging from the water. A lot of people were gasping or yelling or laughing.

Well, as more people exited the water, we saw someone lying face-down in the water, surrounded by a cloud of blood. I am a medic now (I was in school at the time) and have never responded to a water-sustained injury, but this is what I would imagine seeing after a shark attack.

Emergency divers rushed to the water and retrieved a woman, who was wearing only a bikini. She was bleeding from the knee and head. She was barely breathing.

Of course, the scene quickly became chaotic. People were crowding around the medics as they assessed the patient and loaded her on a stretcher. As they moved by me, blood dripped from a bandage placed around the patient's leg.

The rest of the event was delayed, until divers could investigate the scene. They found a large metal object in the water. Apparently, the woman dived and hit the object, knocking herself out.

I saw an article online much later, that said the woman shredded her ligaments and had to undergo surgery for head trauma.

I know a lot of people think events like these could be fun, but during the course of the plunge, two more people had to go to the hospital for complaints of chest pain and arrhythmia brought on by the shock of the cold water, and a few more people sustained minor injuries, such as sprains.

After witnessing the events that day, I enrolled in diving classes so that I could assist law enforcement, and I sometimes assist organizations in exploring water prior to events such as this, to hopefully avoid future accidents.

--J.B.

Minnesota

King of Jingling

Close to midnight, we received a patient between the ages of 3-5 for a foreign body in the esophagus. His parents were arguing with each other—when his mother wasn't crying hysterically, that is.

It wasn't difficult to determine what the child had swallowed. As his father carried him, and with every step his father took, the child jingled.

Yes, the child swallowed a small jingle bell that had come loose from a holiday teddy bear.

We assessed the patient and determined he did not require immediate intervention, but we attempted to keep him still and calm until Endo could assemble an extraction team.

The patient's father interrupted our plans, as we had to scold him several times for singing a song and then attempting to coerce his child into nodding to add a 'beat' to the music. At one point, the father asked a tech if she had any song requests. Dad was eventually asked to stop or remove himself from the emergency room because we were afraid the bell would shift in the child's throat.

Endo prepped the child and extracted the bell with no complications.

--P.T.

Hawaii

Scrooge

At our weekly 'you could just e-mail us this crap so I don't have to come in on my day off' staff meeting, our boss was trying to talk us into donating money for a project he and the higher-ups put together. He wanted each of us to donate at least $20 that would go toward purchasing Christmas decorations to place on headstones at the local cemetery. He wanted to contact the local news and have them do a story, so he could show we were 'giving back' to the community.

He said, "Your donations will allow us to place bells or wreaths around grave markers, so these people know they haven't been forgotten."

I said, "They're dead, so I doubt they care."

The boss (and his boss) didn't find it funny and said I was 'rude to the dead.' I had the choice between donating $30 to their stupid fundraiser, or being stuck on shop cleaning duty for two months. I took the cleaning duty because I cleaned while on-shift, which meant they had to pay me, anyway.

--O.W.

Kentucky

Holiday Hootenanny

This is the story about how I spent last Christmas Eve, my first Christmas and Christmas Eve off in three years.

My sister-in-law is the most obnoxious person in the universe. She is tacky, cheap, and cackles at her own unfunny jokes. I've never really liked her much, and each time my wife invites her over, I think I dislike her a little more. In fact, if I know she's coming over, I try to wiggle out of it or try to disappear to my office for a glass of bourbon. I find whisky allows me to better tolerate her.

My wife *insisted* that I bury the hatchet with my newly-divorced (and Lord knows I have tons of jokes about that, but I won't tell them) in-law, so I was banned from running off to my office, and I was supposed to *try* to behave myself during a family gift exchange.

I wanted to buy my sister-in-law a one-way plane ticket to go back to the Philippines, but my wife used that money to buy her sister a $450 tennis bracelet.

In return, my sister-in-law gave m e a sweater she purchased from an online shop. (Hey, the year before that she gave me a pot of what she calls 'stew,' and I contracted E. Coli, so at least the sweater was a step-up from her trying to poison me.) It was the ugliest sweater of all-time. This itchy wool piece was a gradient of shit-brown and puke-green, and there was an embroidery of what looked like a hippie zombie Jesus on the front, but my wife's sister swore it was supposed to be Santa. I maybe would've bought that explanation if 'Santa' hadn't been embroidered in neon orange and pink thread.

I was about to toss the hideous thing in the fireplace, but my wife of 27-years kindly reminded me that I enjoy sex and would go without it unless I behaved myself and put the sweater on. I came up with every excuse under the sun not to put this godforsaken thing on: contact dermatitis, it's too beautiful to actually wear, someone might take a picture and my taste would forever be judged. I even noted the sweater appeared too small. My wife started taking away sex. I was already down to the next three nights without, so I begrudgingly stood up in front of half our extended family and tried to slip on the sweater. I put my arms in first and then tried to poke my head through the opening.

Like I *said,* the sweater was too small, and my head was stuck. Like, stuck-stuck. Like, "Honey, go get the scissors because we're going to have to cut me out of this thing."

My family thought this was hilarious, seeing me wandering in circles, trying to get this damn shirt off.

As I pulled and pulled and continued wandering, I ran into the curio cabinet and knocked a 10-pound brass vase off the top, which fell on my head and knocked me unconscious. When I fell, I guess my head hit the fireplace hearth. My family had to call 911 and I received four staples to close the gash in my skull. I'm an Emergency Services physician, so I'm sure my coworkers were surprised to see me as a patient that night.

When we got back home, my sister-in-law jumped and latched on for an 'apology hug' as soon as I walked in the door. She knocked me back, and when I fell, I hit my head on the corner of our hall table. I had to return to the ES for three sutures to the other side of my head, and we couldn't get that much blood out of our cream-colored carpet, so I also had to later pay someone $400 to replace our hall carpet.

My wife felt so badly about my injury that she reinstated sex, but I still haven't managed to find a way to drive my sister-in-law away. I guess I should count my blessings now, because next Christmas she'll probably find a way to chop my arm off or set my house on fire.

--K.J., M.D.

Washington, D.C. vicinity

On NYE, I answered a call on our emergency line. The caller requested an ambulance and officers. He said he was injured, after his father-in-law threw a barbequed chicken breast at him. The chicken breast allegedly hit him between the eyes.

I dispatched units to the residence.

The caller was arrested for possession of meth >5 grams, drug paraphernalia, and unlawful possession of a firearm by a felon.

His father-in-law was arrested for battery, but those charges were dropped.

--Z.G.

Michigan

Three Wise Men

Our station was performing at a local elementary school for their pre-Winter Break assembly on the importance of health and fitness. All first responder departments were involved, and we had put together a skit that involved a medic dressed as a clown, a police officer dressed as a 'muscle man,' and I was a firefighter who was supposed to play a coach. I don't even remember what we were thinking when we put this together, but it seemed funny at the time.

I was 'coaching' the police officer in the gym, in front of about 300 kids, parents, and teachers. The guy would pick up a weight and curl it a few times, before I would encourage him to move to the next activity. All the while, in the background, the clown would be mimicking what the muscle man was doing, but he'd 'struggle' with lifting the weight or he would 'fail' at jump roping.

Everyone was having fun, and it was awesome.

Well, the clown picked up one of those elastic toning bands and stood on one end, while 'struggling' to pull the other end of the band toward his upper body. Suddenly, the piece under his foot came loose and whacked him in the nose. Everyone laughed, and we thought it had been part of the skit, so we just kept going.

I 'coached' the cop to pick up another weight and do a few more curls. In the background, the clown was moving slowly. I noticed his eyes were watering, but I couldn't stop the skit to ask if he was okay.

The clown stood behind the muscle man and picked up another 10-pound weight. As he was doing curls, he started using his free hand to wipe tears from under his eyes. I guess he got makeup in his eyes and it irritated his eyesight. He ended up dropping the weight on his foot.

None of these kids knew what was going on, so they all laughed when the clown screamed and stumbled back. We had to abruptly end our skit after the clown tripped over a medicine ball and hit his head on the floor.

Luckily, all the kids still thought everything that had just happened was part of the skit, so we were able to help the medic clown off the gym floor and his partner transported him via ambulance to the emergency room. I guess he fractured his foot, suffered from a concussion, and the makeup that had gotten in his eye burned him somehow, so he had to take time off from work and wear an eyepatch until his wound healed. He told us that the toning band smacking him in the nose was *not* part of the skit.

The school contacted us and said the kids really liked our trio, so we were asked to come back for the school's Springtime assembly. Unfortunately, the medic declined the offer, so we had to find someone else to fill in as our third member.

--N.U.

Illinois

My A&E's 'Top Five' complaints on New Year's Eve:

5.) Alcohol poisoning

4.) Sexual assault

3.) Emergency dental complaints

2.) MVAs

1.) Medical clearances performed for officers

It never fails. EVERY year, idiots come in with cracked, broken, or missing teeth, admitting that they attempted to open alcohol bottles with their mouths. Use a bloody bottle opener, dumbasses.

--M.G.

U.K.

<u>Brain Freeze</u>

I'm a receptionist for an OB-GYN, and last year, about three days before Christmas, I received a phone call that I'll never forget.

The female caller stated she was due at the end of January, but she was hoping she could naturally induce her labor so her baby could be born on Christmas Eve or Christmas Day.

Before I could give this caller my personal opinion or transfer her to a physician or nurse, she told me she had been online, reading ways to induce labor. She wanted to know if 'masturbating with an icicle' really would jump-start labor.

When I asked her why she thought that would induce labor, she told me because the cold would 'startle' the baby and labor would start.

I took her information and placed her on hold.

You should have seen the nurse's face when he got off the phone with her. I've never seen someone look so dumbfounded before.

--T.S.

Wisconsin

<u>O Holy Night</u>

I'm a nurse on our Pediatric Oncology floor and for Christmas, one of my patients received a basketball hoop that we hanged over the door. His ball somehow managed to get stuck in the net, so I (standing tall at 5'2") tried to jump to knock the ball through the net's opening. The cute new doctor was in the room and said he'd get the ball in a minute, but I just *had* to be the hero.

I jumped up for, like, the eleventh time, and felt a sharp pain in my knee. Instead of landing on my feet, I fell back and knocked the doctor over. He got up and tried to help me up. I was laughing so hard that I farted.

My patient yelled out, "Miss Jane, did you just FART? It smells like my dog's fart!"

To add insult to injury, I couldn't even run out of there. I had to go down to the ER, only to learn I had a meniscus tear. I was on crutches for longer than I cared to be, and I had to go to physical therapy. On top of all of that, I learned the doctor I'd been flirting with all weekend was gay. I learned this because his boyfriend was my ER nurse and I had been going on and on about how mortified I was to do this in front of my crush, only to have my nurse tell me they had been dating for two years.

--Initials and location withheld at request

Home for the Holidays

I used to work in a SNF (nursing home), and one of my patients started starving himself after Thanksgiving. It was his way of protesting our facility's 'disgusting' food.

This patient would eat a few saltine crackers each day, but he refused to eat anything from the cafeteria.

Boy, this guy, in his late-80s, threw a huge to-do about our facility's holiday menu. Our cooks were going to serve a 'traditional' dinner, but the menu was altered to serve 'healthy' foods. I could certainly understand this patient's frustration. Instead of ham or turkey, the facility was offering tofu turkey. As an alternative to bread stuffing, management forced the cooks to instead serve Brussel sprouts with chestnuts. Dried cranberries replaced cranberry sauce. The patient said if he only had a few years left, he wasn't going to eat 'cow food,' and he said nobody had a right to tell him he couldn't have steak and potatoes every day, if that's what he wanted.

This patient was so upset about the holiday menu that a week before Christmas, he stopped even eating crackers. He said he'd rather starve to death than eat that 'health nut' food, and he said he missed his home, which had burned to the ground, causing his stay in our facility until his family could work out details with his insurance company.

I was visiting my family and was talking to my mom about the patient. I told her I was concerned for not only his health, but also his emotional wellbeing. I expressed that I didn't know what to do to help the situation, and that I couldn't sneak the man fast food or change the menu at work because neither option was allowed.

On Christmas Day, I had to work, so I wasn't surprised to see that my mom and my Nana had showed up to bring me lunch. We cook in our family, and we may have been accused a few times of going 'overboard' during holidays. My mom and my Nana brought enough food to feed my coworkers and me lunch three times over.

My Nana took me aside and said she wanted to meet the patient I'd been talking about with my mother, so I took her down to the man's room.

Much to my surprise, my Nana had packed two Tupperware containers of ham and roast beef, stuffing, mashed potatoes and gravy, collard greens, cheesecake, and three different flavors of fudge for the man. You would've thought that he'd never eaten before that moment, by the way he gobbled it all up.

What's really weird about all this is that my Nana and my patient started dating.

178

She would come visit him in the facility, and when he was released, they moved in together at a mobile home park for seniors.

--C.W.

Georgia

You can use pinecones for many projects, but I do not recommend using them to masturbate.

Seriously, I spent an hour plucking splinters out of a woman's vaginal cavity because she told me she heard textured objects would enhance her orgasm.

I thought that was the worst shift of the month, until the patient returned. She had developed an infection due to dirt from the pinecone embedding itself in her wounds. *That* was the worst shift of the month.

--R.E., M.D.

Virginia

<u>Wistful Willie</u>

My partner and I were dispatched to a wellness check on our overnight shift. It had been a long night, and from what little dispatch had relayed to us, we both thought the call would be best-suited for law enforcement, but we rarely have the luxury of turning down a call, as in hell freezes over rare.

We didn't really know what we were getting ourselves into. Dispatch said to go to the courthouse and we would 'know' our guy.

When we showed up, we noticed a guy sitting in one of those foldable canvas lawn chairs. He had a beer in one hand and several empty bottles were scattered around him. The closer we got to the man, the heavier the stench of alcohol.

Now, what was really strange about this call is that the man's chair wasn't on the lawn. He was sitting on the iced-over surface of the huge 2-foot-deep wading pool-type fountain in front of the courthouse.

And he was fishing.

Yes, he was fishing from a crudely-drilled hole in the ice.

I was blowing into my hands, trying to stay warm, when my partner blurted out, "What do you think you're doing?"

"Shh!" the man hissed at my partner. "You're going to scare the fish away."

"Sir," I asked, "are you aware of your surroundings right now?"

He took a swig from his beer bottle. "Mm-hmm."

"So," I asked, "you're aware that there are no fish here?"

"Just because others can't catch any, doesn't mean they're not here," he snapped. "Now, go away. You're going to scare them all off."

"Sir," I stated, "you are attempting to catch fish from a pool. I think you should probably head home for the night."

"I think you should shut up and leave me alone before I throw one of these bottles at your face," he retorted.

It was freezing balls out there, but my partner and I decided that we needed to radio for police presence and wait with the man until an officer arrived. Judging by his attitude, we weren't going to be able to convince him to do anything. And if he kept drinking like he was, he would probably pass out and freeze by morning.

Well, some 15-20 minutes later, after this guy really did get so angry about us being there that he threw bottles at us and we retreated to the ambulance, one officer showed up. He had crumbs all over his shirt and when he saw that I was staring, he laughed and said, "Sorry, I wanted to finish my sandwich. It didn't sound too serious."

"It was serious," I said, annoyed. "The guy was throwing beer bottles at us."

I rolled up my pant leg and showed the officer where a bottle had hit me. I was already bruised.

The officer gave me a blank stare and then smirked as he said, "I think you'll live."

"The guy's really drunk," my partner added.

We hung back, and the officer tried to reason with the guy. He even gave the fisherman a chance to leave peacefully, with no charges.

The man responded to the officer as he did to my partner and me.

The officer put his hand on the man's upper arm and said, "Okay, I think you need to spend some time in the drunk tank."

That's when the man threw a punch. He missed the officer's face the first time, but he actually hit the officer with a subsequent punch.

The officer tried to drop the man to the ground, but Mr. Drunky tried to run. In a moment I can only describe as karma, he tripped over one of the beer bottles he'd thrown at us earlier, and he hit the ground.

We had to transport the man to the emergency room because he landed on part of the courthouse's sprinkling system and he poked a hole under his chin. His blood results showed his BAC was .193, a little more than twice the legal limit. The patient was patched up and taken straight to jail. My boss made me file an injury report and be checked out by the ER staff, so I did get to get away from my job for about 30 minutes, while they basically told me what I already knew: I had a bruise and would be fine.

One good thing came of that night. If we hadn't responded to the call, I would have never met my husband…the responding officer (who still tries to cram in time for food when I ask him to do anything around the house).

--W.G.

Location withheld at request

When Winter Comes

M.U. from Nebraska writes:

My grandpa always told us grandkids a story as we were growing up.

He said he was about 19-years-old when a guy in this rural town ran hard on luck and was left homeless.

As the story went, this guy tried to get odd jobs to get by, but few people trusted a stranger on their property, so the man managed by sleeping under porches and eating half-eaten food from trash bins. Grandpa said the man was even known to eat scraps people threw out for their dogs.

Well, the man knew cold weather was coming, and he didn't know how he was going to survive, so he went around town, trying to get himself tossed in jail. He didn't want to break the law, though, so he never got arrested. He was chased out of shops a few times or shooed away from homes, but he felt so badly about disrupting the peace that he just left and tried to think of other ways to get booked.

My grandpa said the guy planned to go to the store and steal something so silly that it wouldn't be missed, but it'd be noticeable to get him in trouble.

I guess the man went to a local dress shop and stole a wire mannequin. He just picked it up from the window display and walked out the door.

While the owner was phoning the police, the owner's daughter followed the man outside and hit him in the back of the head with her wooden-bead necklace. The man tripped over himself when he was hit, and he broke his front tooth when he landed.

The man was arrested and had a place to stay all winter. When he was released from jail, he went to the shop to apologize, and the owner felt that the man's apology was heartfelt, so he offered him a job. The man went on to marry the shop owner's daughter.

Growing up, we just thought it was some random story my grandpa told us. When you're young, you just don't really pay attention to those things.

When my grandpa died, my parents made the now-adult grandchildren help clean out the basement. We found pictures of grandpa working behind the counter at a dress shop, so we finally asked grandma if the story was true. She said it was, and she didn't know the man she busted upside the head was going to be her soulmate.

Tip from the PD:

If you're going to do something illegal, like, maybe throw a NYE party while your parents are out of town, you probably should NOT make a public Facebook page.

Some of the charges from arrests we made at the party: illegal consumption of alcohol by a minor, drug and paraphernalia possession, providing alcohol to minors, disturbing the peace, resisting arrest, public indecency, and public intoxication.

--W.K.

Illinois

<u>2000 Miles</u>

About ten years ago, I was driving my mom's car from Michigan to upstate Colorado. She had just moved there, and she knew I was hurting for money, so she decided she'd pay me to deliver it to her, rather than pay a professional transport company.

I thought my mom would like it if I surprised her by bringing this girl I'd been dating for a few months. I told my mom all about her, but the two had never met.

Well, at the time, I knew this girl was needy. She was one of those high-maintenance girls who complain all the time about everything. We'd fight all the time unless I gave her exactly what she wanted. I was young and dumb and was blinded by how gorgeous she was, so I stayed with her.

We were in the middle of nowhere when I realized we had a flat tire. The drive was bad enough already because the snow was really coming down, even though the weather forecast said it wasn't supposed to snow. So, when I got out of the car and checked the trunk, I freaked out when I saw my mom didn't have a spare. The last town we'd passed was about 20 miles back, and I didn't know how far away the next nearest town was. I tried to use my cell phone, but I didn't have service.

My girlfriend was already bitching because she was 'bored' and she said she definitely wasn't going to be walking in the snow, in the dark, down an empty road in the middle of nowhere. I had to agree with her on that, actually. It was far too cold to go out searching for help, when I had no idea how long it'd take to walk to the town behind us. Luckily, we had about half a tank of gas and there was a half-full gas can in the trunk. I filled up the tank with that and then put the sealed can in the backseat, just in case we needed it again. My plan was to sleep in the car, only running the heat when we absolutely couldn't stand the cold. Of course, my girlfriend bitched about that, too.

I had to pee, so I went to do that and told my girlfriend that I was going to walk a little bit to see if I could pick up cell reception. She complained about being hungry, so I told her I knew my mom kept an emergency kit in the trunk, and it should have energy bars or trail mix.

Because it was so cold outside, I tried to pee by barely unzipping my jeans. I ended up peeing down the front of my jeans. The night couldn't get any worse.

I was maybe about a mile from the car, headed back toward the town we'd passed. I was waving that cell phone around above my head like I was a blind man trying to hit a piñata. Still no reception.

My girlfriend screamed for me, and I ignored her because I was so damn tired already and was pissed off about being stranded in the middle of a damn blizzard that the last thing I wanted to do was deal with her.

When I got tired of her calling to me, I spun around and yelled, "What?"

My mom's car was up in flames. I don't know how I didn't realize it sooner.

When I was running back to the car, I fell and felt my ankle snap. It hurt so bad, but there wasn't anything I could do about it but hobble.

"How did you set the car on fire?" I screamed.

"I found one of those candle things," my girlfriend said. She pouted and said, "I was cold."

"The heat was on," I said.

"But I wanted to smoke, so I rolled down the window. It got cold."

Oh my god.

"Did you drop your cigarette?" I asked. "How did this happen?"

Seriously, at this point, the entire car was on fire. There was no point in even trying to put out the flames because the whole thing was just…gone.

"I told you," she said. "I found one of those candle things in the emergency kit."

"A flare?" I screamed. "You lit a flare? You lit a flare **IN** the car?"

She got mad and yelled at me to stop screaming at her. She really tried to turn it around on me and say it was MY fault that she lit a flare inside the car.

I guess the flare she lit set off a second flare, and then the heat and flames somehow got to the gas can, and the rest was history.

I didn't know what we were going to do. I said something about walking the 20 miles back to that town we'd passed, but my girlfriend refused to go. The thing is, she also refused to stay because she 'was cold and didn't want to be in the dark alone.'

Luckily, someone who lived up a hill in the boonies saw the fire and came down to investigate. This guy had chains on his tires, so I knew he knew what he was doing. He drove about ten minutes ahead of where we were and dropped us off at a sleazy motel. I had to call for an ambulance because my ankle was swollen, hurt like hell, and the skin was so bruised that I looked like a zombie. I broke it.

Now, you'd probably think that there's nothing worse than everything I just told you, but there was something worse.

My mom's insurance had expired the day before, and we didn't know that. Her car was a total loss, and she couldn't even get compensated for it because she'd gotten confused about the due date on her bill. The insurance company wouldn't budge on that, especially after we explained the damages.

The girl I was dating continued to argue that she wasn't responsible for the fire, and she was such a crazy bitch that I broke up with her at the motel. She got mad and took a bus home. I had to stay at the motel for three days, since that's when my brother would be passing through from Detroit to get to my mom's new house.

--D.U.

Michigan

<u>One Special Night</u>

My wife and I are both medics, and if you're involved in a dual-medic relationship, you know finding time off together is virtually unheard of. So, when we managed to get a three-day weekend off together, we were thrilled. We booked a small cabin in this wooded park. It was technically still in our town, but it was different enough from home that we were counting it as a vacation.

The cabins were located probably half a mile apart and were mostly the same inside and out, just small log cabins that had the basic amenities, but no television, cable, or wi-fi. We were far enough out that our cell phone service was spotty. We were cut off from the outside world and loved it.

Each cabin had at least one fireplace and/or a wood-burning stove. Our cabin was beautiful, and during the first hours we were there, we joked about abandoning our 'normal' lives and moving to one of the cabins.

Three days off. Three whole days, and a weekend at that. We really hit the jackpot. Our plan for the weekend was to be as intimate as often as we could muster, sip homemade hot cocoa, and lie in front of the fireplace while we watched the snowstorm swirling outside.

I don't know what time we went to bed that first night. The power went out, so we sat in the dark, drunk off a bottle or two of wine, and eventually we made our way to the cabin's one bedroom.

I do know it was about 03:30 when it happened, because I forgot to shut off an alarm I had set for work, and it went off during the panic.

We weren't awake when the roof collapsed, but we sure were as soon as the roof and snow buried us. The bed snapped from the weight, and I think that's the only reason we didn't die. When the bed fell, logs from the roof created a tent-like alcove. We had to dig our way out of a mound of snow and debris, all while the snow from the storm kept falling. My wife was almost positive she had broken her arm, but she dug anyway.

My wife showed the sense of panic I was trying to hide. I was caught in a rather embarrassing situation: I sleep naked, and our duffle bag was somewhere in that rubble. My wife made me wrap myself in a towel and we chose to go outside because we didn't know if the rest of the structure was compromised.

Outside, I was barefoot on the narrow porch. I was so cold that my 'special buddy' practically crawled back inside me. My wife said we should get in the car and drive until we got cell reception.

As we were walking toward the car, we heard a loud crack. It sounded like lightning striking. Next thing I knew, a tree fell over on our neighboring cabin, and then we heard kids screaming.

Well, I couldn't just let someone suffer, so I told my wife to call for help, and I started running toward the cabin. She had the better idea and said I should drive for help, since I was the one wrapped in a towel. Good plan.

A 5-10-minute drive took about three times longer because of the snow and downed trees along the way. I called 911 on my cell phone and explained the situation. I didn't know if the children we'd heard from the next cabin were injured, how many people were in the cabin, if they were trapped...I didn't know any of that. Dispatch sent four ambulances, two firetrucks, and two squad cars.

I met the first ambulance in the road and they followed me back to the cabins.

I got out of the car and forgot how damn cold it was, so I dropped my towel.

My coworker shot me a strange look and said, "Why are you naked?"

They gave me a jacket and scrub pants to wear. The family from the next cabin over let me wear a pair of the husband's boots. They were a bit too large, but I managed.

Luckily, there were no significant injuries in the cabin park, but when my wife and I returned to work, we learned our guys responded to almost a dozen calls of downed trees or collapsed residences, all thanks to the snowstorm.

My wife thinks we're destined to work ourselves to death and never have a real vacation. I'm starting to agree with her.

--P.L.

Idaho

Extra Work

On a night when all county roads had been closed and the travel service warned drivers to stay indoors unless they were experiencing an emergency, dispatch sent us to a local convenience store. It was 03:30, the snow was piled up outside, I had busted my ass twice because it was my night to salt the sidewalks, and I couldn't sleep, despite being dead-tired. I remember thinking, 'This patient had better be bleeding to death right now.'

The caller was a drunk man who called 911 because his hot dog was too hot and he burned the roof of his mouth. He wanted medical transport, but he had to sit with us while we waited for a tow truck to get us out of the parking lot. During this time, the guy decided his mouth didn't hurt anymore, so he wanted to sign a release.

I was so mad that I could have strangled him. The only thing that was stopping me was knowing I'd have to write a longer report.

--T.V.

Iowa

'Twas the Night

I've been an LEO for years, but the call I responded to on NYE a few years back takes the award for 'wildest call ever,' at least for my career.

We'd been on our feet all night, with complaints of brawls from bars and homes, domestic violence complaints, public intoxication, underage drinking, and of course: noise complaints.

A little after midnight, dispatch sent me to another noise complaint, over in a middle-class subdivision. Several neighbors called to complain that one of their neighbors was having a house party, and they knew the parents were out of town, so everyone wanted us to shut down the party.

I was the first officer on scene, with two additional patrol units on the way, since neighbors complained there were 'way more than 20 people at the house.'

Indeed, there were teenagers crawling all over the property—some quite literally, because they were so drunk they couldn't stand. I saw at least three either half or fully naked teen boys. One kid was wearing a sock on his penis and was passed out on the sidewalk, holding a fire hydrant.

Most of the teenagers, much to my surprise, didn't seem fazed by my presence. Two kids let me inside and another asked me if I wanted to do Jell-O shots with a group of kids in the living room. Beer pong was going on in the dining room, and I witnessed a couple having sex in front of everyone, right there on the laundry room floor. I radioed dispatch and requested additional units.

"We have two more on the way," said dispatch.

"We're probably going to need a few more," I replied.

I was trying to track down the teenager who lived at the residence and was directed to the backyard. In the yard, some kids had a fire going in a metal pit, and another group was over in the corner of the yard, lighting off fireworks.

One kid was naked, completely naked, and was bent over at the waist. He was gripping his ankles with his hands.

And there was a bundle of bottle rockets in his ass crack.

I tried to get to the group before his friend lit the fuses (while another kid was recording on a cell phone), but I wasn't quick enough.

The kid who was using his butt as a launching pad kept screaming and squirming, to the point that the bundle of fireworks dropped to the ground. Some of the kids jumped back. The naked kid stood up and looked around, as if trying to see where the bottle rockets went.

Just seconds later, these bottle rockets started shooting all over the damn place. I put up my arms to keep two of them from shooting my eyes out. One landed on a porch swing and set the cushion on fire when the firework popped. Kids were laughing.

Well, the naked kid stopped laughing as soon as two bottle rockets launched upward and exploded near his testicles. He dropped to the ground like I had tased him, and he was shrieking and crying. I called for medical transport before I approached him. Some of his friends realized I had witnessed everything, so they ran. One guy tried to jump the fence, but his jeans got caught and he fell, knocking a portion of the fence on top of himself. Bottle rockets were still popping off, and the scene was chaotic.

EMS arrived and took naked rocket boy off to the emergency room for second and third-degree burns to his scrotum and surrounding area.

We arrested 18 people from that party, and we had to deploy pepper spray on three others, because they were combative. One kid tried to hit another officer with a metal horse statue. It was wild. I think we had four ambulances out there, and as I was leaving, someone called the fire department out because the garage roof was on fire.

Most of the kids who were arrested received community service and/or probation. All but two of the subjects we arrested were under the age of 18, so they were released to their parents, and most of those parents were hot as hell for having to bail their kids out of jail in the middle of the night. One kid called his mom, but she told him he could sit there all night because she was already in her nightgown and she wasn't leaving the house again until morning. That kid, no joke, he sat in the corner of a cell and he cried the whole night. He even made himself sick a few times because he was crying so hard. I think it was a good life lesson for him, though.

The kid who hosted the party, well, we heard he ended up grounded for the rest of his life, basically. He and his friends did something like $4,000 worth of damage to the home. We heard the dishwasher had been destroyed, the family had to replace the washer and dryer because kids had filled both with vomit and excrement, and I guess the kids locked the family's three dogs in a spare room and the dogs destroyed the carpet. Those were only some of the things we heard happened in the house.

I'll tell you this much: I was known to throw a few parties back in my day, but if I had ever gone to the lengths that this kid did, my parents would have taken turns beating me till I was black and blue, and then I'd be allowed to go two places for as long as I lived under their roof: to school and to take my ass out to the job I'd be working at tirelessly to pay them back for all the damages I made to their home.

--G.M.

Alabama

<u>Warm and Fuzzy</u>

Okay, I'm a female EMT, but I was so embarrassed to respond to this call, mostly because I could understand this lady's own embarrassment.

We arrived on scene around 04:00, for a complaint of 'hygienic accident., chemicals involved.' My partner and I expected someone to have ingested bleach or have had exposure to cleaning solutions.

Not even close.

This woman, who was maybe in her early-thirties, had recently purchased some kind of wax warmer machine. I guess you buy wax beads, put them in a double-boiler-type of pot, then turn on the machine to melt the wax. You can then use a stir stick to apply the wax, which will then harden to form its own 'peeling strip,' eliminating the need for canvas strips.

Well, this woman refused to let my male partner in the restroom. I went in, and I immediately felt uncomfortable. The woman was sitting on the edge of her tub, with bright pink wax hardened to her vaginal area. She had spread the wax around her bikini line, as well as around her labia and between her buttocks.

"I can't pull it off," she cried to me. "It hurts too bad. And now, I don't know how to get it off."

Despite all this, the woman still wanted to go through hair removal.

I basically told the woman I could rip the strips off for her, or I could transport her to the emergency room. She chose a medical transport.

In the end, the lady basically paid $900 for a Brazilian wax, because a nurse told me she went in and ripped the strips off the

woman's bikini area in just a few quick
seconds.

--T.W.

Florida

A Not So Merry Christmas

I'm a dispatcher and took a call from our 911 line from a panicked man. It was the night before Christmas, and he frantically told me he'd sent his kids to hide because there were 'strange men' on his doorstep, who refused to go away.

After taking the man's information, I realized I had two officers on scene already. They were there to take the subject in custody for violating his probation by being identified as someone who'd recently robbed a gas station at gunpoint.

The man on the phone didn't want to hear it, and the situation went from absurd to downright dangerous, when the man started firing shots out his kitchen window.

He continued screaming, demanding I 'call off' the officers because he didn't think he should be arrested, especially on Christmas Eve.

We deployed a tactical team, who apprehended the subject without injuries to the team, himself, or his children.

Officers found two children hiding under kitchen cabinets. They asked officers if the 'bad men' from outside were gone, and they were placed with child services until another family member could be located.

--A.Y.

Illinois

The Gift That Keeps on Giving

Dispatch sent us to a residence after a frantic call of entrapment was reported. We were informed chemicals may have been involved, and that's all we were told.

When we arrived at the trailer, a tearful older woman met us at the front door.

"Can you get it off?" she instantly asked.

"Tell us exactly what happened, Ma'am," calmly instructed my partner.

"Well," she said, "I mixed the plaster, just like it said. Then we did her butt first. While that was hard, we put her on her back and did her titties."

I choked on air and exclaimed, "Huh?"

"It's stuck, and I don't know why. I can't get it off. Like, it's stuck to her, on her butt and titties."

"She's stuck in a plaster cast?" asked my partner.

The woman cried and nodded.

"Where is she?"

The lady pointed to the back of the house. "In the bathroom."

I hadn't said anything for at least a minute already, and I didn't say anything as we moved through the house. I was too blown away at the woman's narrative.

When we entered the bathroom, a woman was lying on her side, with a plaster mold over her breasts that wrapped around just slightly to her back, almost like the cast was giving her a hug. She also had a mold on her buttocks and a portion of her upper thighs. Due to the tightness of the plaster, she couldn't move her upper legs at all. She was nude, with her vagina visible. She had vomited on the floor and it looked like she had dragged herself through it because she had vomit on her arms and elbows. The floor was so gross from mold and dirt that the vomit may have actually cleaned some of the linoleum.

"You barfed?" the older woman asked.

The plaster woman shouted, "I'm scared, okay? I puke when I'm scared!"

I hate vomit. I can mostly handle when I see it already…out, but I get queasy when I see it coming out. I picked a great career for that, huh?

As my partner and I lightly pulled at the plaster, the patient was generally snide and said, "Don't you think that was the first thing we tried?"

Any suggestion we made, she'd shut it down. She called us all the bad names and some that she either made up or were such obscure references that I wouldn't know what they meant. I knew they were bad, though. She called my partner 'Rain Man' so much through the encounter that the nickname stuck at work.

After the older lady started screaming at us, and then the patient yelled at my partner about 9,000 more times, he lost his temper and yelled, "If you didn't want us coming out here to try to get this off, why did you even call us?"

The woman slapped my partner, and he got so mad he told her to 'eff off,' and he went to the ambulance to stew in his anger. Sure, it was unprofessional, but if you had to spend even two minutes with these people, you would have lost your cool, too.

We were doing all we could do. We had tried prying off the mold, tried cutting it with an Exact-O knife, and tried cracking it by banging a piece of wood over a screwdriver like a chisel. The plaster was about three-inches thick. There was nothing we could do. The older woman had neglected to oil the patient's skin prior to applying the plaster, so it was bonded to skin and there was little we could do.

The patient kept refusing medical transport. She said I should be able to remove the plaster for 'all the money her welfare's paying in taxes to pay my salary.' I told her I get paid $9.25 an hour and typically I respond to calls where people are dying, so I didn't have much first-hand experience with people stuck in plaster molds. I tried to say that as nicely as I could, but my patience was wearing thin.

Finally, after an hour of us being there, the woman also lost her patience with our failed attempts to remove the molds, so she demanded we take her to the hospital. I retrieved my partner from the ambulance and we transported her to the ER.

At the hospital, the nurses asked the questions we didn't, mainly: Why the hell do you have plaster on your breasts and buttocks?

Well, the patient's boyfriend was about to go to prison for drug distribution ('and he sold to grownups, not kids, so why should he be arrested for selling to people who could say no?'), so she wanted to make him a mold of 'his favorite parts' of her body for an 'early Christmas present,' since he was at least going away for seven years (the earliest he'd be up for parole). When a nurse commented that the prison probably wouldn't allow the molds, the patient freaked out and spit on the nurse.

We didn't have any calls, so my partner and I stuck around and chitchatted with the ER staff. It was clear they wanted to strangle the patient and the older woman. We discovered the two were related. The patient posted her art project idea on Facebook and her aunt (the older woman) offered to help her, for a small one-time fee of $50 worth of food stamps.

I guess the ER docs had to call all over the hospital to find a cast saw, and it took two-and-a-half hours to remove the plaster molding from the patient's body. She sustained skin tears in the process, but it's better than going through life with a cast on your ass.

--T.M.

North Carolina

<u>Up on the Housetop</u>

Our operator had to go home an hour early because she was having a family emergency, so I was manning the 911 line and the station lines. I figured I only had to do it for an hour, so I wouldn't shoot myself in the foot just yet. It was late at night, too, and nothing was really going on around town, so I was just sitting there, watching football on mute with closed captions that didn't make much sense because it was like the person in charge of the captions also was watching the game on mute and was reporting a failed attempt at lipreading.

A call came through to the 911 line, so I answered and identified myself (it's habit from answering my desk line).

This woman said, "Officer Smith, I need you to send someone out right away."

I asked, "What's your emergency?"

"Well, it's not really my emergency, but there's a raccoon on my neighbor's roof."

I rolled my eyes. We live in a rural location. It's not like we don't see these animals on a daily basis. I'd be more surprised to get a call from someone telling me they hadn't seen a wild animal that day.

"Has it scratched or bitten anyone?" I asked.

"No."

"So, it's just on your neighbor's roof?"

"Yeah."

"You do know this is the emergency line, right?"

"But it's snowing."

"That tends to happen every December."

"What if it gets cold?"

"The raccoon?"

"Yeah."

I laughed.

"I'm serious! I need someone to come out and get it off the roof. It's too cold for animals to be outside."

"Ma'am," I explained, "raccoons live outside. They adapt. Now, I'm going to have to ask you to hang up. This is a line for emergencies only."

The woman huffed and puffed, but she finally hung up.

About five seconds later, the station line rang. It was our non-emergency number. I answered and identified myself.

"Oh," the woman said, "it's you again."

"It's me again," I agreed.

"Well, I need someone to come out here and get a raccoon off my neighbor's roof."

"Ma'am," I sighed.

"What? You said not to call the emergency line, so I called the non-emergency number!"

The only reason the woman hung up this time, is because she said the raccoon ran off someplace. She said she was going to get dressed and go look for it.

I never heard back from the woman, so there's no telling what happened.

--L.A.

Minnesota

The Search

I'm a RN who runs triage in our ED.
Patients see me first, and if they want to be
seen, I assess them and enter their name in
our system. Registration goes to the room
later, to get the rest of the patient's
information.

Well, one night it was snowing heavily,
so we didn't have but maybe two or three
patients over a few hours.

I was at my station, reading a
magazine, when a man walked inside.
This man, and I hate to sound judgmental,
he just seemed like someone you wouldn't
want to be around. His clothes were filthy
and didn't fit. He looked strung out. He
had track marks up and down his arms.
And he was wearing a tank top in the
middle of a snowstorm. He looked lost as
he stood in the lobby.

"Do you need help, sir?" I asked.

He nodded and approached me.

"Do you need to see a doctor?" I asked.

He shook his head. "I know you guys give out free needles to people who are sick, so I need some needles."

He appeared jumpy and I soon realized he was exhibiting symptoms of withdrawal, not a high.

The man fidgeted and pulled a torn scrap of paper from his pocket. He pushed the paper through my window slot and said, "I heard you have to have proof of what you have. That's what I have."

I read a scribbled word off the paper, tried not to laugh, and looked up at him.

"You have rigor mortis?" I asked.

He nodded. "Y-yeah. Can I get some needles now? You know, to help take my medicine?"

I pointed to the waiting room and told the man I'd find someone to help him. I called security and a guard kept the guy busy until the cops arrived.

-M.O.

Maine

Holly Jolly Christmas

We received a patient via EMS for a complaint of 'foreign body in rectum.' A medic already called in report to our unit clerk, who about died laughing. We knew we were about to receive a male patient, mid-40s, with a Santa-shaped holiday candle stuck in his anus. According to the medic calling in report, the patient's elderly mother found him in this 'state,' after she went to the bathroom to learn why her son was sobbing loudly.

I was assigned to this patient.

Lucky me.

When the patient arrived, there indeed was a 10-inch long, 3-inch wide candle protruding from his rectum. The wax had been shellacked, and the candle became suctioned in his cavity. I attempted to pry the candle from the man's rectum, but I couldn't get the piece loosened.

"I didn't do it on purpose," the patient cried.

His mother shushed him and held his hand. "I know you didn't."

"I fell," the patient said.

"I know, baby."

A doctor and his scribe entered the room. The scribe, a shy girl who is usually professional and hardly ever makes a peep, burst into laughter and had to excuse herself from the room.

The doctor and I worked to dislodge the candle from the patient's orifice by using a spreader to widen his cavity in hopes of slipping the candle out.

"What's that smell?" the doctor asked, as we were pulling the candle from the patient's rectum.

That was the most poorly-timed question in history.

I didn't say anything.

"I smell, like, raspberries or something," the doctor continued.

My nose started detecting it, so I nodded and said, "Me, too."

"It's strawberry, actually," the patient mumbled.

"You mean you used the lubricant I found in your room?" his mother yelled. "I thought you said you fell!"

"I did fall!" the patient screamed back, clenching as he yelled.

We had to interrupt the dispute to tell the patient we wouldn't be able to remove the candle if he didn't relax.

As soon as we removed the candle from the patient's cavity, the doctor and I bolted after we told the patient we'd give him and his mother time to 'have their discussion in private.' It wasn't very private, though, because all we did was leave the room and close the curtain. Everyone in the ER could hear the patient's mother screaming at him.

--J.H.

Missouri

We treated a patient for an overdose, and following his three-day stay on ICU, he was arrested.

He wasn't busted for drugs, though.

He picked up the four-foot-tall Christmas tree that was in the ICU lobby and took it with him. Security chased him out an emergency exit, and the cops found the guy in the alley.

--D.W.

Mississippi

Must be Santa

Mental Health Unit Clerk sounding off:

Between November 30-December 31, we experience an overwhelming increase of patients admitted for what our floor likes to call a 'North Pole Complex.'

Mostly, we see patients who believe they are Santa, but I have seen patients who believe they are workshop elves, Mrs. Claus, that they killed Santa, or their purpose in life is to kill Santa.

One year, this guy was brought to our floor after his family signed him in involuntarily. He was adamant that he was Santa's brother, and he believed he should receive compensation from the North Pole because he was a 'celebrity's' sibling. This guy kept everyone up by singing Christmas carols, referenced holiday movies, songs, and folklore constantly, and he told everyone about the injustice of being 'forgotten.'

With that guy, just when I thought things couldn't get any weirder, he escaped from the ER after he was transferred there for a suicide attempt, and security guards found him outside of Lab. He was banging on their service window, demanding a blood test to prove he was Santa's brother.

--S.K.

New Jersey

<u>Did You Not Learn?</u>

I was reading one of your older books and my mates and I were fascinated by a story you recollected, regarding a group of mates who participated in a game of netball with trampolines. Naturally, we decided to try this, and now I want to tell you our results.

We decided to attempt this game after we had sat at a pub for the longer part of three hours. If you have ever known an Australian, you know we do not visit the pub for one pint, so we were smashed when we carried a full trampoline from my neighbor's lawn and his netball ring from his drive. We transported both to the paved roadway.

Rather than run and jump on the trampoline to make a goal, we climbed on the trampoline and attempted to sprint around one another, all while jumping about.

This lasted approximately two minutes, before one of my mates became ill and expelled his sickness. There was vomit everywhere, including on some of us. He then fell off the trampoline and was hanging by his ankle. It was stuck between a metal spring and the outer structure of the trampoline. He became ill again, while he was hanging upside down, and he aspirated on some of his sick, while the remaining sick pooled (up?) his face. He had sick in his eyes and hair.

My mates and I laughed at first, but when we realized there was a medical urgency, we assisted the ill man to his side and one of my mates ran to the neighbor's house. He banged on the door at 04:00 and the neighbor answered the call naked, while holding a golf club. He called 000, and responders arrived.

We were all arrested.

My mate was transported to an ED, and he had to stay for a few days because he broke his ankle and was experiencing respiratory difficulties after essentially inhaling his own sick.

We consume heavily, so I can't promise we will not attempt this again. If we do, however, I hope for much better results.

--D.V.

Australia

How to Deal

I had a rough shift, so I came back to my flat and downed a pint of scotch, before my flat mate asked me to help him with making Christingles. A Christingle is used in many holiday celebrations in our locale and consists of a lit candle inserted into the top of an unpeeled orange, dehydrated fruits and nuts pinned to the orange in four locations by way of skewers, and a ribbon wrapped around the orange. Each component is representative of a religious allegory.

Well, I was certainly in no condition to be making Christingles. I was barely well-enough to stand. But, I tried anyway.

First, I attempted to insert the candle into the top of the orange and squirted myself in the eye with the acidic juice. Trying to rub that out, I fell back against the lit range and set my blouse on fire. My flat mate doused me in soda and inspected me for injuries. I had sustained none and felt horrible about the incident, so I insisted that I remain and assist him in making the Christingles.

I was almost finished with my first piece, when the rest of the alcohol hit my innards and I started to blackout. I fell forward and banged my head on the counter. My flat mate still has pictures of when medics lifted me in the ambulance; I had two wooden toothpicks protruding from my forehead.

The worst part of this is that I'm an A&E nurse. My coworkers had to treat me, and a counselor visited my room to assess my mental state. I had to explain all over again that I was drinking heavily following my shift because one of my patients (a child) had passed as a result of a horrible traffic accident. The counselor suggested to my supervisor that I receive time off to aid in 'emotional healing.'

I still have two dots in my forehead, from where the toothpicks pierced me.

--L.M.

U.K.

Naughty or Nice

Officers, medics, and ER personnel have submitted reasons they've responded to calls or why patients have visited the hospital during holidays. Here are few:

- Domestic dispute over the size of a Christmas tree; noise complaint, no arrests. (L.S., Louisiana)

- Dispute between neighbors, after one neighbor cut down a pine from his neighbor's front yard and used it as the family's Christmas tree, one arrest. (M.M., Washington)

- Patient drank too much eggnog, suffering from indigestion. (R.P., Indiana)

- College professor checked in for abdominal discomfort and diarrhea; his student was arrested after admitting to giving her professor laxative-laced fudge as revenge for giving her a bad grade. (Initials and location withheld at request)

- Dad was piloting child's remote-control airplane, which crash-landed into the child's head; the child required stitches. (N.M., Delaware)

- A family's bull mastiff attacked an intruder on Christmas Eve...the intruder was the man of the house, who dressed as Santa and was sneaking through the back door to surprise his children. (P.M., New Mexico)

- Shoplifting charges to a woman for stealing 32 rolls of wrapping paper; subject was arrested in parking lot. (T.A., Virginia)

- Reports of man dressed in Santa suit groping and flashing women; one arrest. (C.M., New York)

- Reports of man dressed in Santa suit stealing from Salvation Army donation buckets; one arrest. (C.M., New York)

- Reports of man dressed in Santa suit robbing liquor store; no arrests. (C.M., New York)

- Reports of intoxicated man in Santa suit harassing children at playground, attempting to force children to tell him what they wanted for Christmas. Man reportedly gave some children money and candy as 'gifts.' One arrest. (C.M., New York)

- 911 call for 'reindeer damage,' after man captured white-tail doe with tranquilizer. The deer woke up in his home and wreaked havoc until it ran through the sliding glass door and escaped. No arrests, but man scolded on how stupid he was. Conservation Department contacted for follow-up. (Initials and location withheld at request)

- Patient transferred to surgery, following complaint of 'Christmas light bulb' stuck in penis. (A.W., Ohio)

- Patient complaint of 'Christmas ornament stuck in vagina.' Icicle-shaped ornament was extracted, and patient was discharged. (S.U., Wyoming)

- Dog bite to hand, requiring sutures. Owner admitted to forcing dog to pull 'sleigh,' in an attempt to recreate 'How the Grinch Stole Christmas.' (C.A., Kentucky)

- Suicide attempt, with patient stating her boyfriend 'purposely gifted her a 2X shirt because he thought she was that fat.' Boyfriend stated 'he didn't understand women's sizes when he ordered the shirt from a website. She's always complaining that she can't fit in small shirts because her boobs are too big.' (J.J., California)

- Domestic dispute: teenager punched mother for placing feminine pad with eyeball drawn on it inside an 'iPad' box as popular prank. Teenager was arrested and sentenced to juvenile detention center. (Initials and location withheld at request)

Advice from a frustrated M.D.

Do you know how high the numbers are, of patients we treat for papercuts to their tongues during the holidays?

Use a sponge or buy self-adhering envelopes.

Coming to ES because you lick too fast or 'have a nasty taste in your mouth' after sealing too many Christmas card envelopes is not an emergency!

--S.J.-G., M.D.

California

The Mix Up

Last year, on Christmas Day, we received 35 patients in a span of 40 minutes, most of whom arrived via private vehicle. Remarkably, these patients were related. All 35 patients registered for ingestion of poison, and most of them exhibited signs of such: vomiting, pain, chills, lethargy, and more.

We learned the family got together for a holiday dinner, in which a great-great-grandmother prepared most of the foods served. For reasons unknown, the elderly woman kept loose rat poison powder in a Ziploc bag. She had become confused and used the poison in many of her dishes. This was not discovered until another family member went back after realizing people were complaining, and tasted the powder on its own, realizing then it was not flour.

Most of the patients were treated with vitamin K therapy and activated charcoal. However, two patients (a child and an elderly patient) required endotracheal intubation and were admitted to our Intensive Care wing. Both survived.

No charges were filed, as far as I'm aware, as the cook was present in the ER and was ill like everyone else was. We had to administer sedation drugs to her because she was so distraught over her mistake.

--K.E.

Texas

<u>Arts and Crafts</u>

EMS requested police presence at the scene of an overdose. The patient's dealer/brother was at the residence and EMS stated the man was involved in the patient's overdose.

This man voluntarily informed me that yes, he did supply his brother with methamphetamine, and yes, he was involved in producing and distributing the drug to addicts in the neighborhood.

When I moved to place this man under arrest, he was genuinely shocked.

His reasoning?

Well, this man protested his arrest by telling me what he was doing was not illegal. He argued that the drug was made with items he could purchase at the store, so that qualified the meth as a 'homemade product,' and he was simply one of our community's small business owners. He likened his activities to his grandmother's, who purchases yarn from a craft store and then sells her finished products on Etsy.

A judge burst his bubble, and he was sentenced to prison.

His brother, a well-known addict and criminal in our community, entered rehab and has not been in any trouble since his dealer brother was sent away.

--J.C.

Tennessee

A Message to Readers

Thank you for your continued support! I didn't realize how many submissions I received related to holidays. My submissions come as e-mails, DMs on Twitter, or messages on Facebook, so I don't know what I'm getting into until I read each message individually. At times, these messages contain headers in the subject lines that allow me to form an idea of the story, but sorting through submissions is usually a lengthy and emotional process.

I know it seems sudden to have another edition, but I'm one of those introverted 'leave-me-alone' types, so if I'm not writing, I feel like I'm doing nothing productive (and I'm not, really, except sleeping or playing video games). I'm still working on other stuff, but these books allow me to finish something in the meantime.

I have enjoyed interacting with all of you via social media, and I appreciate every review you have left for my books on various websites. Unfortunately, I can't post each one to thank you, but please know I am incredibly grateful and I have personally viewed all reviews. I thank you from the bottom of my heart for your kind words and suggestions.

On that note, I have tried going back to earlier editions to correct typos. I'm unable to do so on several of these editions, as the files have been 'locked' by the publisher and/or distributors. Someone brought to my attention that I typed 'penial' instead of 'penal' in one of my editions, so I guess everyone will have to live with knowing what I must have been thinking about at the time (ha!). I apologize for these errors and can only hope they are small enough that they do not deflect from the books' messages.

257

Most of those books were written after working 8 to 16-hour overnight shifts, when I was trying to unwind before going to bed so I could do it all over again. I guess I didn't take my time to edit them properly, but I now force myself to eye-over work more carefully, so that you receive the best.

To wrap this up, I hope you all have enjoyed this edition. Additionally, no matter where you live/work, no matter what religion you practice or culture you recognize, I wish you all the best. Please remember to be safe in your journeys as you travel for the upcoming holidays. And, most importantly, before you do anything stupid, remember this: you're going to have to explain it to someone.

Have a great day, guys!

Check me out on Twitter!

https://twitter.com/AuthorKerryHamm

My website:

http://www.authorkerryhamm.com

I'm also on Facebook. Drop a search for Author Kerry Hamm to find my page!